Echinacea:
The Immune Herb!

Recycle
Conserve

This book is printed on 60lb recycled paper.

Botanica Press, Santa Cruz, CA

Other books in the "Herbs and Health" series
by Christopher Hobbs:

Milk Thistle—The Liver Herb
Medicinal Mushrooms
Usnea: The Herbal Antibiotic
Natural Liver Therapy
Vitex: The Female Herb
Ginkgo: Elixir of Youth
Foundations of Health
Handbook for Herbal Healing
Valerian—The Relaxing and Sleep Herb
Kombucha: Tea Mushroom

8th Printing, October, 1995
Second Edition

Copyright September, 1990
by Christopher Hobbs

Michael Miovic and
Beth Baugh, copy editors

Illustrations: Christopher Hobbs (Figs. 1B, 3, 5, 6, 7)
Cover photo by Richard Hamilton Smith
Karen Poulos, (Fig.1A)
Mark Johnson (Fig. 4)
Steven Foster (Figs. 8-18)

Botanica Press
10226 Empire Grade
Santa Cruz, CA 95060

TABLE OF CONTENTS

ECHINACEA
THE IMMUNE HERB!

SUMMARY

This booklet presents up-to-date practical information on the use of *echinacea*—an important herb for infections, colds, flu, and a host of other major and minor ailments. Specific instructions are included for the following:

- ✔ Which ailments echinacea works for
- ✔ Choosing the best echinacea products
- ✔ How much to take and for how long
- ✔ Children's dosages

All of this will be backed up with solid scientific evidence, for echinacea is the place where past and present meet, where traditional wisdom and modern research fully agree.

INTRODUCTION

In the 1870's, a doctor in Pawnee City, Nebraska made an unusual challenge to a couple of Eastern doctors. Convinced of the healing power of *echinacea*, an herb he had learned of from local Indians, he offered to let himself be bitten by a rattlesnake and to cure himself with nothing but this plant.   The doctors declined his challenge and lived to regret it. Within a generation, echinacea (pronounced *eke-nay-shuh*) had become the most

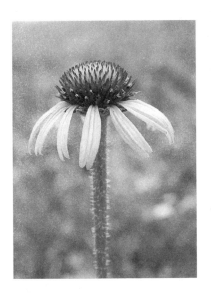

(A) *Echinacea angustifolia*

Shorter ray petals that do not droop. The roots of this species are commonly used. Native to the plains states.

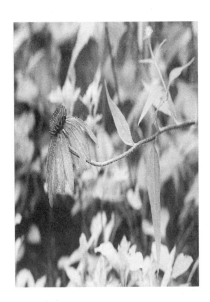

(B) *Echinacea purpurea*

Longer, dark purple ray petals. The tops and roots are used. Native to the eastern U.S. Easy to cultivate in a variety of climates.

Fig. 1   The two main commercial species of echinacea

prescribed herbal medicine in the United States, not only for poisoning, but for a wide range of infectious diseases.

Doctors initially marvelled that a single herb could affect so many different conditions—and without side effects. But echinacea's amazing action was eventually explained with the discovery of the immune system, because the herb strengthens the body's ability to resist infection and poisoning. This

---

The national average is 2.4 colds per year per person—or over 600 million cases in all.

---

has been scientifically confirmed time and again. Since 1930, over 300 journal articles have appeared verifying the effectiveness of echinacea. Today the herb is sold widely throughout Europe and the United States, both in prescription and over-the-counter forms.

Millions of people get colds and flu every year in the United States. The national average is 2.4 colds per year per person—or over 600 million cases in all. Add to this all the other common stresses of modern living—car exhaust, pollution, pesticides, deforestation,

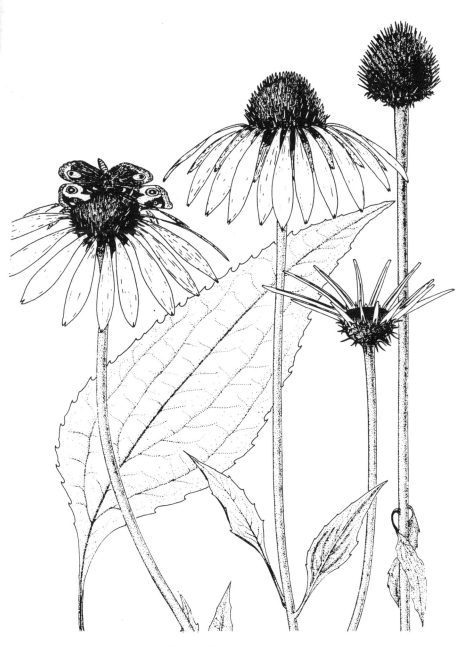

Fig. 2   Echinacea purpurea

chemical wastes from industry, drug-abuse, crime, and plain old fast-living—and you can see why now, more than ever, we need to take good care of our immune systems. There are so many things in our environment today that disrupt the body's age-old processes. Nor can we just down antibiotics forever, because when our immune systems are not working well, antibiotics can only postpone the inevitable.

So if you are intrigued by the possibility of fewer colds and flu, and want to learn about an effective natural alternative to antibiotics for treating skin, gum, and urinary tract infections—to name just a few—then read on! Ten years ago few herbalists in this country had little idea how to use echinacea or even what it was. However, some far-sighted herbalists began importing echinacea products and manufacturing liquid extracts from wildcrafted American herb. Today it is one of the most popular herbs ever, and it is growing more popular as the cold seasons tick by.

THE HISTORY OF ECHINACEA

Echinacea is native to the plains of the United States. It grows wild nowhere else in the world, except for a few sparse patches in southern Canada. So naturally the first people to use this herb were the Native American Indians. Samples of echinacea have been found in archaeological digs of American Indian sites dating back to the 1600's.

The Native American Indians were often skilled herbalists. Of the hundreds of herbs commonly used by the various Indian nations during the 17th and 18th centuries, several stand out. They used ginseng for digestion, golden seal for wounds and infections, sassafras as a spring tonic, slippery elm for soothing the respiratory and digestive tracts, and senega snakeroot for bronchial congestion. These herbs all played an important role in pioneer medicine, and the first four are still in high demand today.

But the Plains Indians revered echinacea above all other herbs and found many uses for it (see Table 1).[2,3] For alleviating toothaches, sore throats, coughs, infections, snakebites and numerous other diseases and afflictions, there was no better medicine. Interestingly, one of the Indians' preferred methods of

---
Table 1

AMERICAN INDIAN USES OF ECHINACEA

TRIBE	AREA	USES
CHEYENNE	Colorado, Kansas	sore mouth, gums, etc.
CHOCTAWS	Mississippi, Alabama	coughs, dyspepsia
COMANCHE	northern Texas	toothache, sore throat
CROW	Montana, Wyoming	colds, toothache, colic
DAKOTA (Oglala)	South Dakota	inflammations
DELAWARE	southern New York	gonorrhea
HIDATSA	—	stimulates energy
KIOWA	southwestern Kansas	coughs, sore throat
MESKWAKI (Fox)	southern Wisconsin	cramps, fits
OMAHA	eastern Nebraska	septic diseases, etc.
OMAHA-PONCA	northern Nebraska	as an eye-wash
PAWNEE	central Nebraska	children's game
SIOUX (Dakota)	northern Nebraska South Dakota	bowels, tonsillitis hydrophobia, sepsis
WINNEBAGO	eastern Wisconsin	anesthetic against heat
---

taking echinacea was to suck on a piece of the root all day. The effectiveness of this practice seems to be corroborated by German researchers who feel that echinacea liquid extracts may begin stimulating immune tissue in the mouth as soon as they are taken.(see fig. 4, p.18)[4]

The Purple Coneflower was known to European botanists as early as the 1690's, and the botanist Moench named the genus *Echinacea* in 1794, from the Greek echinos (sea urchin or hedgehog), referring to the plant's sea urchin-like cone. However, the Europeans knew nothing about echinacea's medicinal properties—or about the properties of any other New World plants for that matter. They had to learn everything from the American Indians, who were quite friendly and willing to share their considerable knowledge with the first pioneers. Books and articles from the early 18th century show that although the settlers brought with them a few herbs (such as plantain), for the most part they had little knowledge of medicinal plants and a great need for them.

"...he offered to come to Cincinnati and.... allow a rattlesnake of our selection to bite him wherever we might prefer.... proposing then to antidote the poison by means of Echinacea only."

But echinacea did not really become renowned until the advent of H.C.F. Meyer, the German lay physician of Pawnee City, Nebraska, mentioned in the introduction. It was Meyer who, around 1870, formulated and began selling a patent medicine containing echinacea (and other herbs such as hops and wormwood) that became quite popular. Meyer unmodestly named his formula "Meyer's Blood Purifier." After sixteen years of experimenting with his preparation, he became thoroughly convinced of its efficacy. He wrote to two eminent medical men of the time, Dr. John King and John Uri Lloyd, and made his now-famous claim that echinacea could cure snakebites.

King and Lloyd belonged to the "Eclectic" school of medicine; that is, they favored the use of herbs in clinical practice. The Eclectic doctors were quite active and influential in the United States from the mid 1800's up through the 1930's. Lloyd later described Meyer's overture as follows:

"In view of our incredulity as to the virtues of the drug in the direction of the bites of poisonous serpents, he offered to come to Cincinnati and, in the presence of a committee selected by ourselves, allow a rattlesnake of our selection to bite him wherever we might prefer the wound to be inflicted, proposing then to antidote the poison by means of Echinacea only. This offer (or rather, challenge) we declined. Dr. Meyer, thinking this was because we had no serpent at our command, again offered not only to come to Cincinnati and submit to the ordeal formerly proposed, but to bring with him a full-sized rattlesnake, possessed of its natural fangs..."[5]

King and Lloyd also dismissed this second offer as quackery, much to their regret. Echinacea was introduced into the materia medica by 1887 and only twenty years later had become the most popular herb among both the Eclectic and regular medical doctors. In fact, it was King and Lloyd who eventually championed the cause of echinacea. Although the herb was always surrounded with controversy, and the American Medical Association never officially accepted it, still many doctors used echinacea faithfully.

The Eclectics used echinacea for many complaints. They employed it as a digestive stimulant and also considered it to be an excellent blood purifier. The plant's immune stimulating properties were first noticed by Unruh around 1914. By then the Eclectics knew that echinacea increased the activity of the *phagocytes*—immune cells that must disarm and recycle bacteria and waste materials in the body. Dr. A. L. Nourse published the following comment in the American Journal of Clinical Medicine in 1914:

"So far as my own experience is concerned, I will state that for conditions requiring strengthening of the reparative forces of the body—raising the opsonic index—I know of no agent of greater value than Echinacea....good for anything requiring the police-powers of the individual to be increased."

The "opsonic index" measures the level of antibodies present in the blood that can render bacteria and other cells susceptible to phagocytosis (engulfment). To be more precise, one could say

Echinacea

(continued on next page)

that the term "blood purifier" signifies a medicine that increases the body's powers of elimination and stimulates immune functions such as phagocytosis.

Dr. Finley Ellingwood, a popular Eclectic doctor and author of the time, had this to say about echinacea:

> "For from twenty to twenty-five years, Echinacea has been passing through the stages of critical experimentation under the observation of several thousand physicians, and its remarkable properties are receiving positive confirmation. As yet, but few disparaging statements have been made. All who use it correctly fall quickly into line as enthusiasts in its praise; the experience of the writer is similar to that of the rest."

Ellingwood recommended echinacea especially for boils, abscesses, pain of breast cancer, poison oak, insect and scorpion bites, tetanus, colds, and urinary tract infections.[6]

Around 1902, echinacea began to gain recognition among the Homeopaths, a school of doctors that believed the axiom that "like cures like." Homeopathic medicines are often given in moderate to high dilution. Under the influence of the Homeopaths, echinacea quickly became popular for general weakness, wounds that would not heal, and as a stimulant for the whole body. It may have been the Homeopaths who introduced echinacea into European medicine, where it has been highly regarded ever since. In the 1930's, German preparations of echinacea became popular, and several of them are still manufactured today.

As the interest in Echinacea has increased, hundreds of scientific studies have been conducted, and numerous medicinal products containing the herb have been made available to the public. Since the early 1930's, the United States has exported over 50,000 pounds of echinacea annually to European markets, and beginning in the late 1970's, herbal manufacturers began making domestic products. Today, nearly every herbal company has one or more echinacea products—it has developed into one of the top-selling herbs of all time.

MODERN VERIFICATION OF TRADITIONAL USES

Pharmacology

In scientific terms, one of the most interesting aspects of herbology is pharmacology—the study of how a given medicinal substance affects the body on a biochemical level. This kind of

the U.S., among both Eclectic and regular medical doctors.
- 1910
Echinacea is recognized as an immune stimulant that increases the attack of white blood cells on bacteria and waste material.
- 1930
Echinacea preparations become popular in Germany.
1930's-1980's
More than 400 scientific journal articles appear exploring the medicinal properties of echinacea. About 50,000 pounds of echinacea are exported annually from the U.S. to European markets.
- 1980
U.S. herbalists "rediscover" echinacea.
- 1986
More than 240 medicinal products in Germany have echinacea as a constituent. In the U.S., echinacea consumption quadruples over previous year and more than 100,000 pounds of the herb are sold.[7]

investigation attracts considerable funding from various commercial enterprises which want to develop and market new medicinal products. Consequently extensive research has been conducted on echinacea. The general conclusion is that it boosts the immune system by increasing the body's ability to ward off, fight, and dispose of bacterial and viral infections. Table 2 summarizes the major physiological effects of echinacea. The information is drawn from over 300 published research papers.

One of the most prevalent uses of echinacea is to forestall or shorten the common cold, flu, and related ailments. Surprisingly, though, few studies have been conducted on this subject, despite the fact that so much research has been done on other aspects of echinacea's activity. It is encouraging that the few studies carried out have given positive results. For instance, in one experiment, 109 children aged 3-5 received a preparation containing echinacea (and 2 other herbs), while 100 did not. The children who received the preparation with echinacea had fewer days of fever and sickness than the control group.[8]

Subsequent controlled studies on children confirmed and amplified these initial results. The same preparation with echinacea proved to be a protective and curative agent for infections of the upper respiratory tract,[9] as well as for viral infections.[10] A similar preparation which contained echinacea and boneset herb demonstrated success in fighting influenza and upper respiratory infections.[11] Of course, it would be more conclusive if the studies were done with echinacea alone, but they can be considered an important step in the study of Echinacea.

Major Active Constituents

The observation of *what* a plant does to the body is one thing, but figuring out exactly *how* it does it can be much more complex. The mechanisms by which pure drug substances cause certain effects are difficult enough to study, sometimes requiring years to pinpoint. Imagine then trying to study an herbal substance, which contains a whole array of different chemical compounds that work together to bring about delicate changes within the body! What researchers have to do is patiently isolate

--------- Table 2 ---------

Echinacea's Major Physiological Effects

- **Stimulates the leukocytes** (white blood cells that help fight infection).

- **Increases "phagocytic power" of the immune cells** (enhances the body's ability to dispose of bacteria, infected and damaged cells, and harmful chemicals).

- **Hyaluronidase inhibition** (this helps protect cells during infection, and prevents pathogens, bacteria, and viruses from entering in the first place).

- **Mild antibiotic effect**

- **Stimulates the growth of healthy, new tissue**

- **Antiphlogistic/anti-inflammatory effect** (helps to reduce soreness, redness, and other symptoms of infection).

- **Stimulates the properdin/complement system** (helps the body control and prevent infections).

- **Stimulates increased production of alpha-1 and alpha-2 gamma globulins** (these prevent viral and other infections).

- **Interferon-like action** (helps prevent and control viral infections).

- **Promotes general cellular immunity**

- **Stimulates killer t-cells**

- **Inhibits tumor growth**

- **Fights viruses**

- **Fights candida** (see following section).

each of these different compounds, called *constituents*, and then test what medicinal effect each has, if any. They also look to see if these constituents are unique to a particular plant or common in many plants, because if a constituent occurs only in one plant, then we can more readily prove that it is this constituent, and no other, which is at least partly responsible for a particular medicinal effect.

Now although some herbalists are not in the least interested in the study of chemical constituents—and indeed one can be a good practitioner without knowing all these scientific details—still, correlating constituents with specific physiological effects has certain benefits. For one thing it expands our general knowledge.

But more importantly, for pragmatic purposes, it helps us to make better herbal preparations. When we know what compounds should be present in an herb, we can determine whether a given sample is the correct herb, and whether it has been grown, processed, and prepared in the best possible way. For while there are many fine manufacturers of herbal products, the sad fact is that with herbs, as with anything else, there are always unscrupulous people who care more about profit than quality. Or, on the other hand, some manufacturers may have good intentions but faulty information about the most up-to-date practices for producing effective medicines or simply be using old, worn-out herbs to begin with. There is an old saying: "garbage in, garbage out."

A tremendous amount of work has been done on the constituents of echinacea. Chemists have isolated scores of compounds, some of them unique to different echinacea species. Often they have also succeeded in linking these compounds with specific physiological effects and activities. Although a full description of this chemistry would be too detailed for a general work such as this one,** for our purposes here we can say that these compounds are divided into two general classes: water-soluble and fat-soluble compounds. Table 3 shows the main

---

**For those interested in a complete review of the chemistry, pharmacology, pharmacy, and extensive history of use of echinacea (including ethnobotany), see my book on the subject, *The Echinacea Handbook* (See reference #2).

types of active compounds found in these two classes for the three major commercial species of echinacea.

Leading researchers feel that both the water-soluble polysaccharides and cichoric acid, as well as the fat-soluble compounds (like isobutylamides and polyacetylenes), boost the body's immune response.[12,13] Professor Wagner, one of the world's leading experts on medicinal plants, believes that the *polysaccharides* (large sugar molecules) are responsible for much of echinacea's immune-potentiating effect.[14] He also believes these compounds stimulate the fibroblasts, inhibit hyaluronidase, and induce interferon—effects which all enhance the body's ability to fight bacterial and viral infections. According to Wagner's theory, the mechanism for these actions would be due to the structure of echinacea's polysaccharides, which greatly resembles that of major compounds in the cell walls of many bacteria. Thus when the body senses the presence of polysaccharides, it may "mistake" them for bacteria and start to build up the immune system. This activity is like an exercise or drill for many immune functions of the body.

However, Rudolph Bauer, an associate of Wagner's, feels that the fat-soluble components of echinacea are more responsible for the plant's remarkable immune activity.[15] It is the isobutylamides of the fat-soluble constituents which give fresh and recently dried echinacea its sharp, tingling taste—that "zing" which some herbalists take as the sign of good echinacea. Although echinacea's polysaccharides do indeed show strong activity, Bauer points out that they may not necessarily be the most important active compounds for a couple of reasons. First of all, compounds very similar to echinacea's polysaccharides are found in a wide range of plants, especially in the daisy family. Second, polysaccharides may be broken down in the digestive tract before they can even be absorbed into the blood.

Of course, it is conceivable that immune stimulation may take place in the mouth, where immune tissue is activated immediately by contact with polysaccharides. However, this theory in turn is disputed, since the alcohol in tinctures may destroy the potency of echinacea's polysaccharides.

Table 3			
The Active Compounds of Echinacea			
Fraction	**E. purpurea**	**E. angustifolia**	**E.pallida**
Oil-soluble	Isobutylamides	Isobutylamides	Polyacetylenes
Water-soluble	Cichoric Acid Polysaccharides	Echinacoside Polysaccharides	Echinacoside Cynarin

As you can see, like so many other things in life, we do not yet know everything there is to know about echinacea's active ingredients—but we do know enough to create excellent and consistent echinacea products right now.

Echinacea preparations have a solid track record in clinical and laboratory studies, and thousands of doctors currently use them for a long list of infectious diseases.

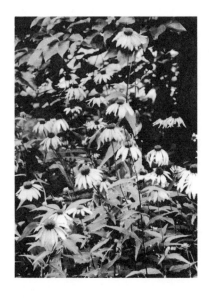

Fig. 3   Echinacea purpurea

A patch of wild plants growing in the garden.

WHAT CONDITIONS IS ECHINACEA BEST FOR?

This is, naturally, the practical question that most readers will want answered, and it is a good question. As it turns out, echinacea is ideal for what is called in Traditional Chinese Medicine "surface conditions," that is, illnesses that come and go and are not deeply seated or chronic. Colds and flu are classic examples of surface conditions, as are abscesses, bronchitis, sore throats, and many other common infections, if they are not chronic. For such conditions our immune systems have cells called *macrophages* (this means, literally, "big eaters") that quickly migrate to the site of infections to stop bacteria, viruses, and other pathogens from gaining a foothold, or to eliminate them once they have already entered into the body. Tests show that echinacea greatly stimulates these macrophages and increases their effectiveness. (see fig. 4, p.18)[16,17,18]

I have found that children respond especially well to echinacea.

Another very important use of echinacea is for candidiasis. Recent controlled studies demonstrated that a fresh liquid preparation of echinacea, taken orally, caused a marked reduction in recurrences of candidal colpitis and/or vulvitis (vaginal yeast infection).[19]

Table 4 lists the major conditions for which echinacea has been clinically tested and found to be effective. Herbalists, acupuncturists, chiropractors, naturopaths, medical doctors, and other health practitioners commonly use echinacea to treat these ailments. Be sure to review them carefully, since there was not room to list them all in the text. Also, be sure to review the accompanying Table 5, which explains the dosages suggested for treating each of the conditions in Table 4.

The only thing I can add is that the overwhelming consensus of my own experience plus the testimony of friends, patients, and acquaintances, is that proper and regular use of echinacea can be effective for most of these conditions, especially when combined with rest, a high-quality diet and other healthy habits. I have also found that children respond especially well to echinacea.

However, my research and experience indicate that echinacea may not be the herb of choice for long-term or profound immune deficiencies, such as cancer, AIDS, or chronic fatigue syndrome (Epstein-Barr virus). In both Traditional Chinese Medicine (TCM) and Ayurveda (a traditional system of medicine from India), it is known that surface conditions are treated with one class of herbal formulas and profoundly deficient states with another.[20] Herbs such as *Astragalus membranaceous, Ligustrum lucidum, Panax ginseng*, and many fungi (especially reishi, *Ganoderma lucidum*) are used in these latter cases.[21,22,23] I call them "bone-marrow reserve" or "deep defense" builders and correlate them with the TCM concept of "Wei Chi tonics" or "protective vitality" builders. Echinacea can be used in conjunction with these other herbs for deeper-acting tonic formulas. (see fig. 4, p.18)

A good example of the difference between the surface and deep immune system was highlighted in a German study with children who were undergoing radiation and chemotherapy for cancer. One side-effect of drug and radiation treatment is the severe reduction of the white blood cell count, which is unfortunate since it is precisely white blood cells which must fight the spread of cancer. In this study, the researchers were happy to find that an echinacea preparation helped restore the white blood cell count in most of the children. However, they also noted that a few of the children did *not* respond to the echinacea preparation because their immune systems were too depleted on a deep level. In other words, they had no more "bone marrow reserve" (all of our immunologically-active cells originate in the bone marrow). Happily the echinacea eventually worked once the children were allowed to rest for a long time to nourish their bone-marrow reserves.[24] There is mounting evidence that the bone-marrow reserve builders mentioned above can help the bone marrow to create more immune fighters.[25]

One of the most important uses for echinacea seems to be to forestall or shorten the common cold, flu, and related ailments.

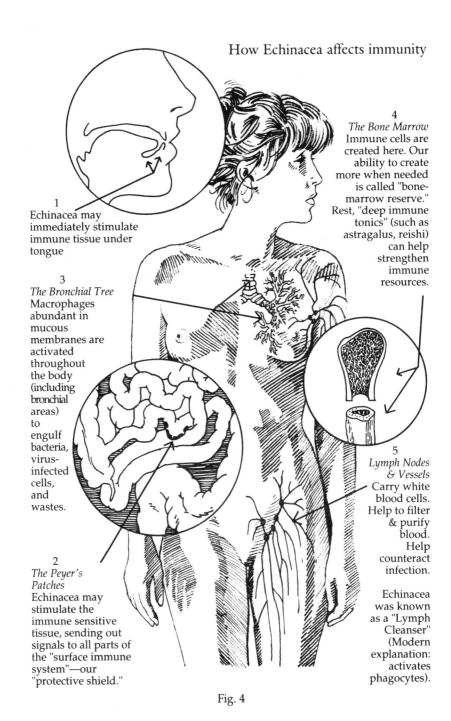

How Echinacea affects immunity

4
The Bone Marrow
Immune cells are created here. Our ability to create more when needed is called "bone-marrow reserve." Rest, "deep immune tonics" (such as astragalus, reishi) can help strengthen immune resources.

1
Echinacea may immediately stimulate immune tissue under tongue

3
The Bronchial Tree
Macrophages abundant in mucous membranes are activated throughout the body (including bronchial areas) to engulf bacteria, virus-infected cells, and wastes.

5
Lymph Nodes & Vessels
Carry white blood cells. Help to filter & purify blood. Help counteract infection.

Echinacea was known as a "Lymph Cleanser" (Modern explanation: activates phagocytes).

2
The Peyer's Patches
Echinacea may stimulate the immune sensitive tissue, sending out signals to all parts of the "surface immune system"—our "protective shield."

Fig. 4

Table 4

Main Uses of Echinacea

General infections and wound healing	use echinacea topically and internally (see table 5); internally add garlic
Colds or flu	especially before onset or in early stages, take a *protective* dose (see Table 5 for dosage guidelines). Take a *full course* when experiencing aggravated symptoms; if desired, put drops in ginger tea or sage and lemon peel tea
Candidiasis	for an acute situation, take a *full course*; for long-term use (up to several months), a *tonic dose;* add black walnut, garlic and pau d'arco
Strep throat	use *full course* as a gargle, then swallow solution combined with usnea liquid extract;[26] add propolis
Staph infections (impetigo, under nails,etc.)	take *protective dose* internally; apply locally full strength with usnea liquid extract
Urinary tract infections	for cystitis and urethritis especially, take a *full course,* as needed, followed by *maintenance dose* for 2 weeks; put drops in a tea of marshmallow root, licorice and pipsissewa; add usnea

---

Pelvic Inflammatory Disease (P.I.D.)	*full course* at *maximum dose,* stop for 3 days, then take another course as needed; *maintenance dose* for up to a month; rest and a nourishing diet are essential; do sitz baths daily
Tonsil and non-strep throat infections	use *protective dose* as a gargle, then swallow solution; use drops in sage tea; add usnea
Upper respiratory tract infections	put diluted solution of tea or tincture in nasal spray bottle and spray on back of throat several times a day; take *full course* internally; may use with grindelia and yerba santa herb or extract
Infected wounds	keep area moist with tincture, full strength; take internally; may use with comfrey poultice externally
Burns	*use maintenance dose* topically and internally; may be used with calendula cream
Herpes	use commercial creams or full-strength tincture topically; internally use a *protective dose* during acute phases, and a *tonic dose* thereafter, especially during times of stress

Skin ulcers	keep the area moist with tincture (full strength)
Psoriasis	*take maintenance dose* internally, and apply externally; add milk thistle extract internally
Whooping cough	*full course* during acute phases. For children under 5, reduce dose to 10 drops 3-5x/day; for ages 6-10, 20 drops 3-5x/day: for 11-16, 1 dropperful 3-5 x/day; may add drops in thyme tea with a little goldenseal
Bronchitis	take *full course* internally; may add grindelia andyerba santa or add to elecampane (¹/₂), marshmallow (1) and licorice (¹/₄) parts
Leucopenia (low leucocyte count) and low t-helper cell levels	take *full course*; however, this treatment works only for leucopenia due to radiation therapy and other causes not directly related to long-term deficiency of immune function and general nutrition, malabsorption, or abusive life-style; astragalus, codonopsis, ligustrum and reishi tea or commercial product can be taken concurrently for up to 9 months for deeper immune strengthening

Rheumatoid arthritis	take *tonic dose* for anti-inflammatory effect; try taking a feverfew tablet everyday (see my article for more information)[27]
Allergies	take *tonic dose* for food allergies, environmental sensitivity, hay fever, and any other allergies not related to long-term immune deficiency; can be used with goldenseal and eyebright tea or extract
Toothaches and mouth and gum infections	gargle and swish extract, then swallow; apply full-strength to infected area 3-5 times daily; may add propolis or myrrh liquid extract
Bites and stings (insects, animals—rattlesnakes)	apply full strength on the bite and take internally
Blood and food poisoning	take large doses internally (1-4 droppersfull, or 4 capsules, every 2 hours)
Boils, carbuncles, abscesses	apply externally, and take *full course* internally
Eczema	use *maintenance dose* internally; may use with *Viola tricolor* liquid extract

HOW TO USE ECHINACEA

When taking Echinacea for the first time, always start with a low dose for a few days, to assure that there is no individual sensitivity. Then the dose can be gradually increased to full dose.

Table 5		
Suggested Dose Schedule		
Type of Dose	**Quantity**	**Duration**
Tonic Dose	10 drops/day of tincture 2 capsules/day 1 tablet/day	up to 9 months, as needed
Maintenance Dose	20 drops 2X/day of tincture 2 capsules 2X/day 1 tablet 2X/day	up to 2 months
Protective Dose	1 dropperful 2-3 X/day 2 capsules 3-4X/day 2 tablets 2X/day	10 days on, 4 days off, for up to 3 cycles
Full Course	1-2 droppersful every 2 hrs. 3-4 capsules every 2 hrs. 1-2 tablets every 2 hrs.	10 days maximum, then use protective dose
Children's Dose	under 6: 10 drops max/dose 7-10: 20 drops max/dose 11-13: 30 drops max/dose 14-16: 1 dropperful max/dose	same as above, depending on severity of the condition

There are good reasons to assume that echinacea works best during a ten-day course. German researchers have found that the stimulation of phagocytosis (one important parameter of immune activation) lasts only 10 days, both with oral doses and when injected.[28,29] After this time, the immune system may become accustomed to large doses—and at least the enhanced phagocytosis, an important aspect of blood purification, drops to just above normal. This corresponds with my own experience. Interestingly, the German researchers found that the maximum immune stimulation came between 3 to 6 days after the first dose was taken. In other words, echinacea may take at least one day before it "kicks in." That is why it is best to begin taking it immediately when one feels a cold or flu (or any other infection) "coming on."

I believe that this research suggests three things.

1) Take large doses of echinacea only when needed, not as a matter of course.
2) Take small 10-15 drop doses (per day) of echinacea for up to 9 months to "exercise" the surface immune function or "protective shield."
3) If large doses are required over a longer period than 10 days, try taking the echinacea in cycles—10 days on and 5 days off.

It has been my experience that it is important to keep taking echinacea for 48 hours after the symptoms of a cold, flu or infection disappear—or a relapse may occur.

For external application, use echinacea salve or ointment (available commercially); or apply the liquid extract to a cotton pad and fix it in place; or make a tea of the root or leaves and apply in a similar fashion. Be sure to change the dressing often for acute infections.

The above conditions are ones that the author has either seen echinacea work for first-hand, or in a few cases they are ones commonly treated with echinacea by eclectic or German doctors. However, no herbal remedy will work for everyone 100% of the time. Also, any natural remedy works better when combined with healthy habits.

IS ECHINACEA SAFE?

This is the next question that people usually ask, and the answer is overwhelmingly Yes. Tests performed on *E. purpurea* have demonstrated it to be completely non-toxic and nonmutagenic.[30] That is the beauty of this natural antibiotic. In my personal experience, I have found no side effects during seven years of regularly taking a 50% water and alcohol extract of fresh *E. angustifolia* roots. Once I took a full ounce of the preparation at one time. However, I have heard several reports of minor skin rashes resulting from use of the tincture,[31] and one report concerning throat irritation from drinking the tincture straight from the bottle. (This can be counteracted by diluting the tincture in water or other liquid before taking a dose, especially for children.)

WHAT IS THE BEST KIND OF ECHINACEA PREPARATION?

There are four major kinds of echinacea preparations that are commonly available.

1. Raw plant (whole, powdered, or "cut and sifted")
2. Liquid extracts, or tinctures
3. Powdered extracts
4. Products that contain echinacea in combination with other herbs (such as golden seal).

All of these can be of high quality, provided one knows how to choose them. The key questions one should keep in mind when selecting any echinacea products from the shelves of herb stores, natural foods stores, or other sources, are the following:

> ✔ What species of echinacea, or combination of species, does the product contain?
> ✔ What is the quality of the herbs contained in the product?
> ✔ How is the product prepared?

The Species of Echinacea

Although there are nine different species of echinacea that grow wild in this country (all east of the Rockies), only three have a history of use and clinical testing. Hence only these three are commonly sold in health food stores and herb shops: *Echinacea angustifolia* (narrow-leaved coneflower), *Echinacea purpurea* (purple coneflower), and *Echinacea pallida* (pale coneflower). Refer to Table 6 and figures 1A, 3 and 6 to help you distinguish between these species.

Naturally people often ask me which of these three main species is the best to use. After reviewing the world's literature and using several different species myself for many years, I feel that *E. angustifolia* and *E. purpurea* are equally beneficial.

Table 6

The Main Species of Echinacea[32]

Species	Appearance
Echinacea purpurea	tall and stout, with wide leaves; large purple flowers with a high (1-2") cone; yellow pollen; grows scattered in eastern states
Echinacea pallida	smaller, with narrow leaves; pale purple petals; white pollen; grows in northern plains states
Echinacea angustifolia	shortest plant, with narrow leaves; shorter petals, not so drooping; grows in middle to lower plains states

Echinacea angustifolia roots have a long history of use by John Uri Lloyd, the first echinacea product manufacturer in this country. He made a success of a high-alcohol, highly concentrated liquid extract called "Echafolta". This preparation had many years of effective use by doctors in the early 1900's.

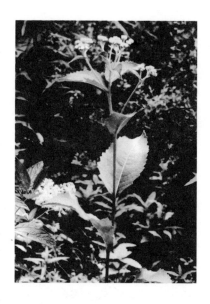

Fig. 5 *Parthenuim integrifoluim*

A common adulterant of Echinacea purpurea, known as "prairie dock."

But *E. purpurea* has a great track record, too. Dr. Gerhard Madaus began manufacturing a liquid from the tops of this plant, when seeds he received from America turned out to be the wrong kind. He was expecting *E. angustifolia*, and was thus disappointed, but later found that *E. purpurea* worked quite well in its own right.

As for *E. pallida*, it is often sold as *E. angustifolia*, both in this country and in Europe. According to Dr. Bauer, probably the world's leading authority on the chemistry of echinacea, *E. pallida* has immune-stimulating properties, but some of its important constituents may break down faster than in the other species, and its roots contain fewer of the important immune active amides.[33] Among herbalists there seems to be a consensus that *E. pallida* works, though it is not as desirable as the other two.

Steven Foster, author of *Echinacea Exalted*[34]—an informative book well worth getting for those interested in further study—has this to say about the matter:

E. pallida* is, "Traditionally not considered as good as the other 2 species of echinacea."

When I asked him what he thought about *E. angustifola* and *E. purpurea* having higher concentrations of the amides, he answered,

> "It's clear that the efficacy of *Echinacea* is not due to a single active component. Besides, much of what has been sold as *E. angustifolia* is in fact *E. pallida*, which is a highly variable plant. Until a great deal more clearly defined research is conducted, any conclusions on *E. pallida* are subjective generalities at best."

The conclusion seems to be, "keep an open mind," though Foster did say that *E. angustifolia* was his own personal favorite among the three species. When I asked him why, he answered, "I like the flavor."

Basically, the fresher the echinacea, the better it is.

Today, the best-studied preparations of echinacea are liquid concentrates of the tops of *E. purpurea*. Some say this is no coincidence, since E. purpurea is by far the easiest species to cultivate and gives the highest yields. Thus perhaps the other species make just as good medicine, but simply haven't been studied as much. Still, because *E. angustifolia* was the preferred species in this country for many years—first by the Eclectics and later by various herbalists—many modern manufacturers mix the roots of *E. angustifolia* with the tops of *E. purpurea*. This makes for a more complete blend. Some companies even add the seeds or flowers of either species, probably because the seeds give a biting, tingling taste to the preparation which has often been taken as a sign of high quality herb.

What this all means, in pragmatic terms, is that when buying echinacea products, you want to be sure that you are getting pure *E. angustifolia* **and** *E. purpurea*, not other species of echinacea or even completely different herbs. Recently I worked closely with an analytical laboratory in testing many of the commercially available echinacea products for purity, and we found that supposed *E. angustifolia* products often contained a mixture of *E. angustifolia* and *E. pallida*.[35] And the situation with *E. purpurea* was even worse—it was commonly adulterated with *Parthenium*, a plant that is not even a species of echinacea and has little medicinal value! Thus it is a good idea to buy only "Certified Organically Grown" echinacea, because it is almost guaranteed not to be adulterated.**

Wild vs. Cultivated Species

A subcategory of the discussion about which species of echinacea to use concerns the question of whether the wild or cultivated species are better. The widespread rumor that wild echinacea is stronger than its cultivated counterpart is precisely

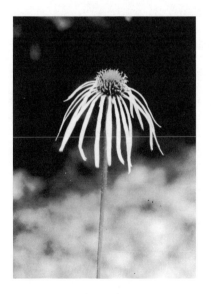

Fig. 6 *Echinacea pallida*

A common adulterant of "wildcrafted" *E. angustifolia*.

**The problem of adulteration is widespread, but not hopeless. The rise of small, family-owned enterprises dealing in certified organic or wildcrafted herbs during the last decade has helped create a quality-consciousness in the industry. Also, the American Herbal Products Association (AHPA) recently forged a tentative accord among members who are manufacturers and distributors to stop selling adulterated products.

that—nothing more than a rumor. There is not an ounce of clinical or laboratory evidence to support this claim. In fact, there is every reason to believe that carefully grown organic echinacea will be of a more consistent quality than wild echinacea that happens to grow in poor soil or is subjected to adverse weather conditions. Also, as our knowledge of the chemistry and pharmacology of echinacea grows, it is not inconceivable that someday we may, with breeding techniques, be able to create more potent strains of echinacea. These kinds of innovations over "the wild" have already had spectacular results with wheat, rice, corn, and other major food crops.

If you buy certified organic products.....the herb is grown in living rather than lifeless, sterile or devitalized soil.

The truth of the matter is that there are some very compelling reasons *not* to buy wild echinacea—one of the main ones being to preserve our wilderness. For the last 100 years (or so) wildcrafters have been digging between 50-100,000 pounds of echinacea annually for exportation to Europe—and this may be a conservative estimate. I have heard that there are still vast fields of wild echinacea in places, but, considering that the plant's native range land has mostly been destroyed, developed, or over-grazed, it seems likely that these wild populations will soon be endangered. For instance, one species of echinacea, *E. tennesseensis,* was considered extinct until a small population was discovered in an open cedar glade in Davidson County, Tennessee.[36] For this reason I strongly encourage organic, commercial cultivation not just of echinacea but of most medicinal plants and use only organically cultivated echinacea (both *E. purpurea* and *E. angustifolia*) in my own formulas.

Another good and practical reason to avoid wild echinacea is that the government does not regulate the wildcrafting industry very well; hence there is no legal guarantee of any kind for the label "wild." Many products are sold that claim to be "wild *E. purpurea*," which is impossible, because *E. purpurea* grows too sparsely to be collected from the wild. It is all commercially cultivated in the western United States and in Europe.

If you buy certified organic products, on the other hand, you can be sure that the herb is grown in living, rather than lifeless, sterile or devitalized soil, and that no pesticides or herbicides were used (these, ironically, may suppress the immune function). Products that contain organic echinacea are not much more expensive than products that do not contain it, and often they cost the same. Guidelines for using the name "organic" or "certified organic" vary from state to state, but a national law is imminent and may soon be a reality.

How to Determine Quality

Basically, the fresher the echinacea, the better it is. Some manufacturers go to great lengths to preserve freshness—they will even make liquid or powdered extracts of the plants right from the field. It has been known for a long time that echinacea roots lose their potency when exposed to air, warmth, or moisture for more than a few months (in some cases exposure even for weeks is enough to ruin the herb). This is especially true of the cut or powdered herb. Thus, if you buy bulk echinacea from an herb store, make sure to buy the whole root instead of the powdered

---

Dried whole root retains its active properties very well.

---

herb, or at least large pieces of the root. Powdered herb in capsules or tablets can also degrade (because both plastic bottles and gelatin capsules breathe), though obviously less quickly than bulk powder. Capsules packed in glass bottles last longer than those packed in plastic ones.

Table 7	
Expected Shelf Life for Echinacea	
Preparation	**Shelf Life**
Whole leaf	1/2 to 1 year
Whole root	1 to 2 years
Cut and sifted root	1 year
Powdered herb, capsules	1 to 1 1/2 years
Powdered herb, coated tablets	1 to 2 years
Powdered extract, capsules	1 1/2 to 2 years
Liquid extract (tincture)	2 to 3 years

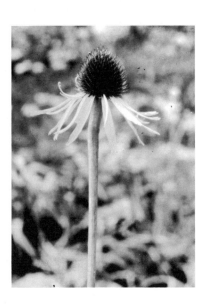

Fig. 7 *Echinacea parodoxa*

The only yellow-flowered Echinacea. Not sold commercially, unless as an adulterant of wildcrafted *E. angustifolia*.

Of course, there are always pros and cons. Two good reasons to buy capsules are that they are convenient and cost-effective. So if you do opt for capsules, look at the *manufacture* date (not the expiration date) stamped on the bottle. Try to buy bottles that are as recent as possible and never more than one year old. If a bottle has no date on it, it is better not to buy it since there is no way to know how old the herb is. If you can only find the

Echinacea

Table 8

The Pros and Cons of Echinacea Preparations

Preparation	Advantages	Disadvantages
Whole root or herb	holds freshness for over a year, if stored properly; cost effective	must be ground or powdered before use; less convenient
Cut and sifted	ready for making tea; cost effective	loses quality faster than whole root; less convenient than patent products
Capsules or tablets of powdered root	convenient; cost effective	best to use before 1 1/2 years; not as concentrated
Freeze-dried preparations	preserves freshness	can absorb moisture; shelf-life may be reduced[38,39]
Liquid extracts (tinctures)	hold quality for over 2 years; convenient; fairly cost effective; work fast	some people object to alcohol; glycerin can be irritating if not diluted
Powdered or concentrated extract	potent; convenient; no taste when in capsule or tablet	not so cost effective; not as quick-acting as liquids

expiration date, ask the store owner or call the manufacturer to find out how long the expiration date is from the date of manufacture, and do your math!

The most durable type of echinacea preparation is liquid extracts or *tinctures*. These retain their potency for up to two or even three years, especially when stored in amber bottles, away from heat and light. The main drawback of tinctures, however, is that their alcohol content may irritate or not be acceptable to some people. In this case the drops can be highly diluted in water or juice or placed in boiled water to evaporate much of the alcohol. Table 7 shows the normal shelf life, in my experience, for the major commercial preparations of echinacea (assuming favorable storage temperature, low light levels, and normal humidity), and Table 8 lists the general pros and cons of the major commercial preparations of echinacea.

How the Product is Prepared

This issue concerns the more technical aspects of the factors that contribute to quality discussed above; it is not as critical to the average consumer, though it may be of interest.

...we do not yet know everything there is to know about echinacea preparations. Even if there is a "golden recipe" to be discovered, it may well be many years before we find it.

Bauer found that dried whole root of echinacea retains its active properties very well—much better than powder.[37] However, because of the amount of cellulose and lignin present in the whole root, a concentrated extract may be more effective in the amounts generally recommended with commercial preparations (1-3 capsules or tablets, 2-3 X/day). Apparently the extraction process also releases constituents from cell walls, which may make extracted preparations more assimilable by the digestive tract. But, on the other hand, we do not yet know that sensitive constituents are not lost due to the heat of the extraction process itself. For this reason, most herbalists feel that the best preparations use as little heat as possible for the extraction process—pluses for cold-processed tinctures, freeze-dried and shade-dried preparations.

In simple language, all this just means that we do not yet know everything there is to know about echinacea preparations. Even if there is a "golden recipe" to be discovered, it may well be many years before we find it. In the meantime, when all is said and done, it is my experience that if the herb used is of good quality, and if it is processed soon after harvest, then the product will be effective. The details of what ratio of ethanol-to-water is best; whether dried, freeze-dried, or fresh herb is best; and whether *E. purpurea*, *E. angustifolia*, *E. pallida*, or some other untested species is best—all of these questions may well be fine-tuning.

Growing Echinacea

Find seeds or small plants of echinacea in a nursery and grow them yourself. *Echinacea purpurea* is the easiest to grow. It will do well in nearly any climate, but does not prefer hot, dry areas. If you live in such a climate, grow the plants in partial shade, or keep them well-watered. *E. angustifolia*, a native to the plains, prefers hot summers and very cold winters. I have found that *E. angustifolia* does not do as well as *E. purpurea* in a coastal climate. *E. pallida* is not as fussy as *E. angustifolia*, and it grows more quickly and vigorously.

The easiest way to grow echinacea is to buy the plant already in a pot, which can be set out in rich, well-drained soil and mulched with compost. The tops of *E. purpurea* can be harvested throughout the summer; try eating a leaf daily as a mild immune "tonic"—the flavor is provocative and you might even like it!

The roots of any of the three species can be dug in the fall around the first freeze, after the tops have died back. Wash them and dry them well in a warm, shaded place with good air circulation and store whole for future use. For detailed information on the fine details of growing echinacea, including commercial cultivation, see my book *The Echinacea Handbook*.

By growing this beautiful plant, we are helping to preserve our precious wild resources and getting to know the plant first-hand— herbs always seem to work best this way.

A FEW COMMENTS BY HERBALISTS
WHO USE ECHINACEA

Ed Smith (Herbalist, Manufacturer, Williams, OR):

"Because of its potentiating effects on the body's immune system, Echinacea favorably influences a broad array of medical maladies and can often bring about rapid and complete healing where all else seems to fail.

No remedy, herbal or otherwise, *always* works, but I can say that in all my years of dispensing medicinal herbs, I have never seen an herb work as effectively, consistently and safely as Echinacea. It is *the* herb to convert the most ardent herbal skeptic."

Cascade Anderson Geller (Clinical Herbalist, Portland, OR):

"It is important to warm up echinacea—add a warming, stimulating agent in formulas, especially when used for acute infections; ginger, cayenne, cinnamon or prickly ash—my favorite because it's a native American plant. With some people it can have no effect in acute cases after taking large amounts, but it works best in combination with other herbs. Add golden seal and warming herbs, especially with mucous membranes (colds & flu).

Student case studies in the naturopathic clinic show that a combination works better."

Brian Weissbuch (Clinical Herbalist, San Anselmo, CA):

"Echinacea's primary indication is lymphatic stasis with inflammation and immune-depression. As exposure to environmental pollution increases, this herb becomes increasingly valuable. Bear in mind that universal panaceas are mythical creatures—echinacea is not for everyone."

Amanda McQuade (Clinical Herbalist, Santa Rosa, CA):

"Echinacea is deserving of its old name, prairie doctor. I couldn't imagine not having it as a core of my herbal practice.

So I am encouraging all my clients to grow it, as the wild sources are being overpicked, to address our society's burgeoning interest in immune health, for which echinacea is a blessing from the earth."

Michael Tierra (Clinical Herbalist, Author of Way of Herbs):

"As a native perennial of the Great Plains, it is the very symbol of North American herbalism beginning with its use by the Native Plains Indians and continuing with the great Eclectic herb movement of the late 19th and early 20th centuries.

Energetically, echinacea has a cool energy with a bitter, pungent, slightly sweet flavor. From a Chinese medical perspective, it goes to the lungs and stomach which rule the "wei chi" (immune system) and the liver which is the organ of detoxification. It therefore is classified and used in the Chinese herb category of clearing heat and detoxifying.

Echinacea's prime area of effect is for hypermetabolic conditions of "damp heat", especially when there is yellowish pus. Being a cool, detoxyifying herb it has less value for conditions and constitutions that arise out of deficiency and internal coldness, as in the case of whitish or clear discharges. Therefore, one may not expect echinacea to work alone either in conditions of yin deficiency (auto-inflammatory, wasting diseases), or in mild conditions arising from internal coldness or low metabolism.

All parts of the plant are effective but the root should be preferred in cases which tend towards deficiency, while the aerial parts are effective for conditions which tend more toward excess."

Brigitte Mars (Herbalist, Alfalfa's Market, Boulder, CO):

"Echinacea is truly one of nature's important gifts. I have seen this herb help thousands of people avoid the overuse of antibiotics. There have been few, if any, side-effects and many health benefits. This is a plant we need to grow more of. It seems like people come into the store for the first time just for this one product."

Appendix 1

Comprehensive Literature Review

The second section of this book (the appendix) is intended for more technically-minded readers. Here I present detailed, scientific information on the botany, chemistry, pharmacology, toxicology, and clinical uses of echinacea.

Knowledge about many of the popular medicinal plants from North America in common use today derives from the Native Americans. Many tribes had thousands of years of direct experience with herbs. In their culture, and in later early American-European culture, several of these herbs are of special interest—but especially herbs from the genus indigenous only to North America, *Echinacea.*

Samples of Echinacea have been found in archeological digs of Lakota Sioux village sites from the 1600s (Wedel, 1936). Echinacea has experienced cycles of increased popularity in the time it has been known to the European-based settlers, from the turn of the 19th century.

Currently there is a reawakened interest in echinacea in the United States. The last few years have seen a tremendous rise in popularity from relative obscurity between 1930 and 1980 partly due to increased interest in immune system functions. Echinacea is probably one of the most promising immune strengtheners and modulators, with numerous scientific studies and rich clinical evidence in its favor. Over the last 99 years, various echinacea species have had over 400 journal articles to their credit.

Twenty years after its "discovery" by the lay doctor H. C. F. Meyer and introduction into the Materia Medica by the Eclectic doctor John King and John Uri Lloyd (ca. 1887), it had become the number one herb in popularity among both Eclectic and Regular medical doctors. Although orthodox medicine officially refused to recognize its worth and it was surrounded by controversy, many physicians used it, defending its efficacy. The centennial of its "discovery" by the medical profession comes at a time when its popularity has never been greater.

BOTANY

Origin of The Names and Taxonomy

Echinacea is one of the coneflowers, a group of native American wildflowers from the Daisy Family (Asteraceae) characterized by spiny flowering heads, with an elevated receptacle which forms the "cone." Other genera in this group, the Heliantheae, the largest tribe in the Asteraceae, include *Rudbeckia* L., *Ratibida* Raf., and *Dracopis* Cass. (Stuessy, 1977). However, newer work has resulted in the placement of Echinacea in another tribe, the *Ecliptinae*, while the other three genera were placed into a new subtribe, *Rudbeckiinae* (Robinson, 1981).

Echinacea has only a few common names in English. The most widely encountered common name is Purple Coneflower, for obvious reasons. One also sees Purple Kansas Coneflower, Black Sampson, Red Sunflower, Comb Flower, Cock Up Hat, Missouri Snakeroot and Indian Head (Lyons 1907). *Echinacea purpurea* (L.) Moench has been popular in American horticulture as a border plant or as a plant in wild gardens for many years. A number of cultivars have been selected, varying in flower size and color, among other characteristics. Some of the more popular include Brightling, Golden, Queen, Leuchstern, Masterpiece, Rosequeen, Scarletta, The King (Bright crimson rays of good substance), The Pilot, Winchmore Hill, and Sombrero (bushier and with larger crimson-purple rays) (Kelsey, 1942; Dress, 1961).

A number of Latin names have been used for the plants now accepted as being from the genus *Echinacea*. The Purple Coneflower was known to European botanists as early as the 1690s and may have been first collected in Virginia (and sent to European botanists) by the Reverend John Banister in 1680-2 (Morison, 1699). In his *Plantarum Historiae Universalis Oxoniensis* (part 3), Robert Morison, the first Professor of Botany at Oxford University, calls the Purple Coneflower "Bite of the Devil" and gives it the first "official" name: *Dracunculus virginianus latifolius, petalis florum longissimis purpurascentibus*, which roughly translated means, "The Little Dragon of Virginia, having flowers with long, reddish-purple petals projecting out to the side."

Other botanists (e.g., Herman, Catesby, Dillenius, and Clayton) described the plant in the early 18th century, but it was Linnaeus (1753), the great Swedish botanist and physician, who named the Purple Coneflower, *Rudbeckia purpurea* (=*Echinacea purpurea*), after Olaf Rudbeck, a fellow botanist and physician. This name was used in the botanical and horticultural literature as late as 1860 and is even occasionally found in contemporary literature.

Today, the purple coneflowers are placed in the *genus Echinacea,* first described by Moench (1794). This name replaced *Brauneria,* previously used by de Necker in 1790 (Britton, 1896), but later discredited. Table 9 summarizes the origin and first descriptions of all nine currently accepted Echinacea species.

The most complete recent taxonomic treatment of the *genus Echinacea* is the work of Ronald L. McGregor from the University of Kansas (1968). He describes several varieties and includes data on chromosome numbers, comparative anatomy, and hybridization among Echinacea species. Hybridization and chromosome work may be important in the future in the development of more effective strains for medicinal use. The chromosome number can affect the amount of secondary compounds that a plant produces, and populations with preferred chromosome numbers may be found in the wild, or developed, to be used in the manufacture of botanical medicines.

Because *E. pallida* is still confused with *E. angustifolia* in commercial trade, exact chemical and morphological criteria for distinguishing samples in commerce have been worked out by Bauer, Heubl, and others (Heubl *et al.*, 1988; Heubl & Bauer, 1990).

DESCRIPTION

Plants from the genus Echinacea are herbaceous perennials whose stems are simple or branched, upright, and ascend from either a vertical taproot *(Echinacea angustifolia)* or branched, more fibrous roots (*E. purpurea*). The plants are either glaucous (waxy) and smooth, or variously hairy, usually with coarse hairs. The leaves are petiolate (stalked) below, becoming sessile (stalkless) and smaller above, and are prominently 3-5 veined, either ovate, ovate lanceolate, elliptical and coarsely toothed or entire.

The flowering heads are single at the end of the stems or branches, having both ray and disc flowers, of which a prominent characteristic is the conical or hemispheric "cone" of the receptacle. The phyllaries (subtending bracts of the head) are in 3-4 series, imbricated (overlapping), the outer ones more leaf-like, lance-shaped to lance-linear, transitioning into the receptacle spines (called pales). These exceed the flowers in length (a key character and genus trait) and end in sharp or blunt spines. The ray flowers are sterile, in one series, strap-shaped, 2- or 3-notched at the end, sometimes reflexed characteristically downward, usually rose-colored or purple, sometimes white or yellow (*Echinacea paradoxa* (Norton) Britton) to red. The disc flowers are fertile, the corolla expanding below into a fleshy bulb-like base, while the tube is cylindrical and has a 5-lobed erect limb. The achenes (seeds) are 4-angled, 3-3.5 mm long, and the pappus consists of a short, smooth or toothed crown. McGregor's key to the species can be found in his original paper (1968) and is reprinted in *The Echinacea Handbook* (Hobbs, 1989). See this work and Foster (1991) for more complete information on the botany and taxonomy of the genus.

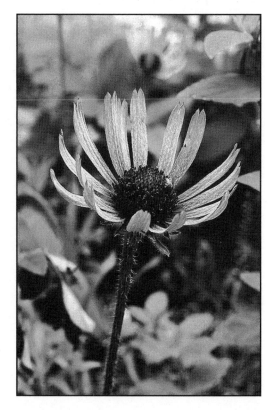

Fig. 8 Tennessee Coneflower (*Echinacea tennesseensis*). Photo © 1993 Steven Foster

HISTORY OF USE

Ethnobotany

Many Native American tribes had a substantial pharmacopoeia, and some used herbs and other internal medicines extensively. In the early days of European colonization of the North American continent, native peoples were known to share their considerable skill with the Europeans (Vogel, 1970), who generally were in need of medicines, due to the difficulty of transporting official drugs across the Atlantic. Of all the indigenous medicines introduced by Native Americans, echinacea may be one of the most important.

According to Gilmore (1911, 1913), "Echinacea seems to have been used as a remedy for more ailments than any other plant." Meyer, the German lay physician who first introduced echinacea to the medical profession, learned of its healing virtues from Native Americans (possibly the Pawnee or Omaha) living in Nebraska at the time. Table 1 lists all the tribal uses reported in the literature. For a thorough review of the ethnobotany of echinacea, see Hobbs (1989) and Foster (1991).

Most of the information we have on the ethnobotany of Echinacea comes from tribes that roamed the great plains region.

Early European-American and Eclectic Uses

Little mention was made of echinacea in medical literature before H. F. C. Meyer, a lay doctor from Nebraska, "discovered" the virtues of *E. angustifolia* around the 1870s and began making a patent medicine from it.

The earliest reference to the medicinal uses of any of the species of Echinacea appeared in the second edition of *Flora Virginica*, by L. T. Gronovius (1762), derived from the notes of John Clayton (1693-1773), an English botanist who lived in Virginia for 40 years. Clayton states that *E. purpurea* "bears a sharp-tasting root and is very valuable in treating the saddle-sores of horses" (Berkeley & Berkeley 1963). Rafinesque (1830) mentions that the Sioux used Echinacea for syphilis, and Riddell (1835) notes of *E. purpurea*, "root thick, black, very pungent to the taste; aromatic and carminative, little known." Comings (1847), in perhaps the first journal article on echinacea, says that "the tincture or decoction is a specific for the venereal disease in its worst forms, having never been perseveringly employed without success." The noted American botanist, Asa Gray, wrote in his *Manual of Botany* (1848) that *E.*

purpurea has a "root thick, black, very pungent to the taste, used in popular medicine under the name of black sampson." He later said that it was "called black sampson by quack doctors" (Gray, 1879).

The Eclectics

The Eclectics, prominent in the United States from 1845 to the 1930s, were a group of medical doctors who employed botanical medicine extensively in their practices. In their heyday they maintained a number of medical schools in various parts of the United States—most notably in Cincinnati—and claimed practitioners in every part of the country.

The Eclectic school was a major force in bringing Echinacea to the forefront of herbal medicine. John King, one of the best-known Eclectic doctors and author of the important *American Dispensatory* (1852), together with John Uri Lloyd, an eminent pharmacist, writer, and manufacturer, was instrumental in introducing Echinacea to the medical profession in 1887. The history of the introduction of *E. angustifolia* into mainstream medicine has been quoted widely; the best accounts are Lloyd's own *History of Echinacea angustifolia* (1904), and the Lloyd brother's *A Treatise on Echinacea* (1917).

At first King and Lloyd were incredulous, because Meyer, the German lay doctor who sent the plant to them, made such exaggerated claims of its miraculous healing powers, most of which were too wild to be believed. They ended up taking back their words after reluctantly trying it, and echinacea eventually became the most popular herb of the entire Eclectic era.

The Eclectics used Lloyd's famous *Echafolta*, a clear, high-alcohol preparation, as well as his "Specific Medicine Echinacea," in addition to commercial products from many other drug companies, such as Merck, Wyeth, and Parke, Davis. These preparations were recommended for a wide range of ailments, many of which involved anti-microbial and anti-toxin effects. Specifically, its virtues were extolled for insect bites, snake and spider bites, the bites of rabid dogs, diphtheria, typhoid, carbuncles, cerebro-spinal meningitis complicated by herpes, blood-poisoning, puerperal septicemia, gonorrhea, eczema, syphilis, and pyemia (King & Meyer, 1887; Hobbs, 1989). Unruh (1915) even foreshadowed our current knowledge of the action of echinacea as an immune stimulant, using it in a manner to treat tuberculosis, reporting that it increased the phagocytic powers of the leukocytes, similar to vaccines.

The Regulars

The "regular" medical establishment at the time openly criticized the use of echinacea (Chamberlin, 1905; Couch & Giltner, 1921a, b), and the *Journal of the American Medical Association* ran articles that declared it a useless "quack remedy." Meanwhile, as a number of official organizations were criticizing it, many physicians were using it in clinical practice and extolling its virtues (Thackeray, 1923; Editorial, 1930), and ironically, it was included in the 1916 United States *National Formulary*, an inclusion which lasted until 1950. Reports by doctors in the medical literature of the time show that successes were seen with puerperal fever "where all else fails," teeth and gum disease, boils, typhoid, anthrax, and even in veterinary practice (Webster, 1891). For a comprehensive review of the medical articles see Hobbs (1989) and Foster (1991).

CHEMISTRY

History of Chemical Analysis

It is fitting that the first published report on the chemical constituents of Echinacea was by John Uri Lloyd, in 1897. Before that time, 11 years after its introduction into general medical practice, little was known of its chemical makeup. References were made only that it was at first "sweet," and then "acrid." This in itself says something about its chemistry, for we could surmise that the root might contain sugars and perhaps essential oil, which it does. The methods of assay were crude, however, as was evidenced by Couch and Giltner's study (1921a, 1921b). They had no idea at that time the depth of Echinacea's chemical profile and physiological activity.

Despite the crude methods available to him, Lloyd was thorough in his investigation of *E. angustifolia* and submitted it to extensive tests. After completing his analysis, he reported that "echinacea contains minute traces of a colorless alkaloid...." Although it is likely that other compounds, besides alkaloids, may have been responsible for Lloyd's positive alkaloid test (Bauer, 1992), a German research team (Röder, *et al.*), detected traces (.0065 in dried roots) of the pyrrolizidine alkaloids tussilagin and isotussilagin in *E. purpurea* and *E. angustifolia*.

Today a great deal more is known about the chemical makeup of various Echinacea species, thanks to a number of groups working in

Germany, particularly to Professor H. Wagner and his students at the Institute of Pharmaceutical Biology in Munich. One of the researchers, Rudi Bauer, has done a tremendous amount of work to legitimize the popular and medical uses of the genus. Although there is undoubtedly more to learn about the active constituents of echinacea, we do know that among the many compounds that have been already identified, the alkylamides, cichoric acid derivatives, polysaccharides and possibly glycoproteins are the most promising. Other major groups of compounds that have been found in various echinacea species include flavonoids, monoterpenes, a number of caffeic acid derivatives, hydrocarbons such as N-alkanes, polyacetylenes, high molecular-weight polysaccharides, and traces of pyrrolizidine alkaloids.

For a more complete review of the past and present investigations on the chemistry of *Echinacea* species, see Bauer and Wagner (1990, 1991) or Hobbs (1989).

Note: Analytical work (circa 1955 to 1987) on *E. angustifolia* must be called into question, because of possible misidentification of the species. It is possible that *E. angustifolia* could have actually been *E. pallida* (which, however, was also official in the *National Formulary* (1916-1946)), or even other species that were not clearly differentiated by early researchers. Early work on *E. angustifolia* in Germany could have also been *E. pallida*, and any work on commercial *E. purpurea* roots (not *E. purpurea* tops or work on the product Echinacin®, where the plants were grown by the manufacturer) could have actually been performed on *Parthenium integrifolium*, a common adulterant after about 1910 (along with *Eryngium aquaticum* and *Lespedeza capitata*). Work that falls into this category is marked as such in the following table, which reviews the chemistry and pharmacology of echinacea species (Moser, 1910; Lloyd, 1917).

For an explanation of immunological terms, see page 75.

The Chemistry and Pharmacology of Echinacea Species

Species Key: EA=*E. angustifolia*, EP=*E. purpurea*, EPA=*E. pallida*, ET=*E. tennesseensis*, ES=*E. simulata*, EPX=*E. paradoxa*, EAT=*E. atrorubens*

Constituent	Species	Reported Activity	References
Carbohydrates			
Sucrose, levulose	EA (EPA?)		Heyl & Hart, 1915
Pentosans	EA (EPA?)		Heyl & Staley, 1914
Fructose	EA,EP	fructose of the roots lowest in May, higher in Summer and Fall	
Polysaccharides			
Inulin storage (fructans)	EA (EPA?)	5.9% in EA roots beneficial to diabetics; -inulin activate compliment, inulin in EP, EA occur in much higher concentration in the fall and winter than spring-summer, and tinctures contain quantities of fructans up to a polymerization of DP 15	Heyl & Staley, 1914 Kraemer & Sollenberger 1911 Giger & Baumann, 1989
Hetero-polysaccharides (structural) (PS)	EA,EPA,EP	Two high molecular weight PS were characterized which showed macrophage-stimulating activity. The same or similar PS have shown weak antihyaluronidase activity.	Wagner & Proksch, 1981 Wagner & Proksch, 1985 Bonadeo *et al.*, 1971
Phenolic compounds			
Caffeic acid derivatives		this class of compounds can be used to identify EA, EP,EPA	Bauer & Wagner, 1991
Echinacoside	EA EPA ES,EPX,EAT	weak antibiotic activity	Stoll *et al.*, 1950 Becker *et al.*, 1982 Bauer *et al.*, 1987 Bauer *et al.*, 1991b
Verbascoside	EA,EPA	aerial parts only	Bauer, *et al.*, 1988a
Des-rhamnosyl-verbascoside	EPA	—	Cheminat, *et al.*, 1988
6-0-caffeoyl-echinacoside	EPA	roots only	Cheminat, *et al.*, 1988
3-malonylglucoside			Cheminat, *et al.*,1989
Cynarin	EA,ET	roots only	Bauer & Wagner, 1987
Chicoric acid	EP,	most in EP flowers, roots; immune-stimulating	Becker *et al.*, 1985 Jurcic, *et al.*, 1989
Caftaric acid &	EP,EPA	mainly aerial parts	Bauer *et al.*, 1988a
Chlorogenic	EA,EPA	leaves and stems	Bauer *et al.*, 1988a

Constituent	Species	Reported Activity	References
Isochlorogenic acid	EA,EPA	—	Cheminat, *et al.,* 1988

Flavonoids

Constituent	Species	Reported Activity	References
Misc.	EA(EPA?)	from the leaves: luteolin (L), kaempferol (K), quercetin (Q), Quercetagetin-7-glu, L-7-glu, K-3-glu, Q-3-ara, Q-3-gal, Q-3-xyl, Q-3-glu, K-3-rut, rutoside, isorhamnetin-3-rut	Malonga-Makosi, 1983
Misc.	EP	Q, Q-7-glu, K-3-monolycoside, K-3-rut, rutin, Q-3-rob, Q-3-xylosylgalactoside, 2 diglycosides of isorhamnetin	Malonga-Makosi, 1983
Quercetin	EP,EA	EP, 0.48%; EA (EPA?), 0.38%	Malonga-Mak., 1983 Bauer, *et al.,* 1988a
Rutoside	EA,EP,EPA	main flavonoid in the leaves	

Fatty Acids

Constituent	Species	Reported Activity	References
		—	Heyl & Hart, 1915
Linoleic, oleic, scerotic & palmitic acids	EA(EPA?), EP		Heinzer *et al.,* 1988

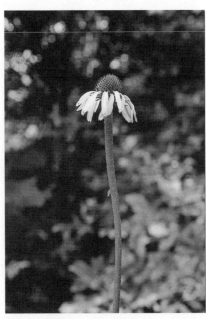

Fig. 9 *Echinacea atrorubens.*

Constituent	Species	Reported Activity	References
Alkylamides biosynthesized from oleic acid			
Echinacein	EA	dry root contains 0.0004-0.01%; shows insecticidal activity (toxic to houseflies) stimulates the flow of saliva (sialagogue), local anaesthetic (leads to the famous tingling effect of echinacea products); recent tests have not found echinacein in either EA or EP, thus, the above-mentioned effects may be due to other isobutylamides	Jacobson, 1954, 1967 Bauer & Wagner, 1991 Greger, 1988
Misc.	EA,EP	numerous alkylamides characterized from all species tested (only traces in EPA); they probably play an important role in echinacea's immune-stimulating activity; the pattern of alkylamides in EA and EP are noticeably different, making them excellent markers for identification and stan-dardization; they occur in the highest concentra-tions in flowers and roots:	Bohlmann & Grenz, 1966 Bohlmann & Hoffman, 1983 Bauer *et al.*, 1989c Remiger, 1989 Bauer *et al.*, 1988a Verelis, 1978 Bauer & Wagner, 1991
	EA	rt, 0.009-0.151; lv, 0.001-0.03%	Bauer & Remiger, 1989b
	EP	rt, 0.004-0.039%; lv,	
	EPA	traces	
	ET	similar pattern to EA	
Essential Oil	EP	dried leaves, 0.64%; flowers, 0.56%; roots, 0.24% maximum	Schindler, 1953
	EA	flowers & leaves, <0.1%	Heinzer *et al.*, 1988 Bos, *et al.*, 1988
	EPA	roots, 0.1-4.0 highest in April and May; leaves, <0.1%	Neugebauer, 1949 Heinzer *et al.*, 1988

Essential Oil Components of Echinacea Species

EA (EP?)
2-methyltetradeca-5,12-diene — Woods, 1930
2-methyltetradeca-6,12-diene

Constituent	Species	Reported Activity	References
penta-1,8Z-diene 1-pentadecene		—	Voaden & Jacobson, 1972
Pentadeca-8Z-en-2-one			Schulte *et al.*, 1967
Echinolone		promising juvenile insect hormone activity	Jacobson *et al.*, 1975
Humulene			Becker, 1982
EPA Pentadeca-8Z-en-2-one Pentadeca-8Z,11Z-dien-2-one Pentadeca-8Z,13Z-dien-11-yn-2-one Tetradeca-8Z-en-11,13-diyn-2-one		main components of root oil	Heinzer *et al.*, 1988 Bauer & *Wagner*, 1987
EP Caryophyllene 2.1% Humulene 0.6% Caryophyllene epoxide 1.3% dodeca-2,4-dien-1-yl-isovalerate		major components of root oil	Becker, 1982 Martin, 1985
Vanillin		aerial parts	Bohlmann & Hoffmann, 1983
p-hydroxycinnamic acid methyl ester Germacrene D Germacrene alcohol		roots and aerial parts essential oil of the fresh plant only	Heinzer *et al.*, 1988 Bauer *et al.*, 1988b
EA,EPA,EP above-ground parts Borneol, bornylacetate, pentadeca-8-en-2-one, germacrene D, caryophyllene, caryophyllene epoxide			Bos, *et al.*,1988
EA,EPA,EP seeds alpha-pinene, beta-pinene, beta-farnesene, myrcene, limonene, carvomenthene, caryophyllene, germacrene D, epishiobunol, 1,8-pentadecadiene			Schulthess *et al.*, 1988
Hydrocarbons N-alkanes	EA (EPA?)	a series C10 to C33 in leaves and shoots	Verelis & Becker, 1977
polyacetylenes	EA,EP		

A number of polyacetylenes have been identified from EA, EP, (EPA?) EPX, ES, and EAT. They are somewhat species-specific, which means they may hold promise for species identification in raw material, but not commercial products, because they are readily oxidized by atmospheric oxygen and have mostly been absent in tested commercial products.

Schulte *et al.*, 1967
Bauer *et al.*, 1988e.

Constituent	Species	Reported Activity	References
Alkaloids			
Tussilagin	EA,EP	0.006% in dried root	Röder *et al.*, 1984
Isotussilagin	EA,EP	these pyrrolizidine alkaloids do not contain a 1,2-unsaturated necine ring system, which must be present to confer liver toxicity for this class	
Miscellaneous Compounds			
Betaine hydrochloride	EA (EPA?)	—	Heyl & Hart, 1915
Glycine betaine	EP	—	Soicke *et al.*, 1988
Phytosterols	EA	in leaves, stems: beta-sitosterol, stigmasterol, sitosterol-3-*B*-*0*-glucoside	Verelis, 1978
n-triacontanol	EA	in leaves and stems and	Verelis, 1978
behenic acid ethyl ester	EA	in roots	Verelis, 1978
Misc. compounds	EP	methyl-*p*-hydroxycinnamate, 13-hydroxyoctadeca-9Z,11E, 15Z-trienoic acid, labdane derivative	Bohlmann & Hoffmann, 1983
Cyanidins	EP,EPA	cyanidin-3-*0*-B-D-glycopyranoside, cyanidin-3-*0*-6-malonyl-B-D-glycopyranoside	Cheminat *et al.*, 1989
Glycoproteins	EP3	3 were identified (associated with the cell-wall fraction); many glycoproteins are immune-activating; EP glycoproteins inhibit antigen-antibody reactions and are reported to be antigen specific *in vitro*	Beuscher & Kopanski, 1987
			Egert & Beuscher, 1992

Mineral & Vitamin Content of Echinacea spp.

Mineral	Ion mg/100 g Crude root
Aluminum	129 mg
Calcium	776 mg
Chlorine	76 mg
Iron	48 mg
Magnesium	117 mg
Potassium	314 mg
(Coulter, 1930)	

Vitamin Content

Vitamin C   0.214% in fresh *E. purpurea* blossoms by dry weight
(Gunther, 1952)

Other Species

Echinacea simulata
Tests reported by Bauer and Foster showed that this plant contains ketoalkenynes as in *E. pallida*, alkamides the same as in *E. angustifolia* and echinacoside (Bauer & Foster, 1991).

Echinacea paradoxa
Chemical analysis of this species revealed a number of ketoalkenynes and other constituents that are almost identical as *E. pallida* (Bauer and Foster, 1991).

Echinacea tennesseenis
HPLC analysis of cultivated roots revealed that *E. tennesseensis* may have a closer taxonomic relationship to *E. angustifolia* than previously realised, by having eight alkamides in the nonpolar fraction as well as cynarine from the polar fraction in common. The two species also lack ketoalkenynes, but it is interesting that only *E. tennesseensis* lacks echinacoside (Bauer, *et al.* 1990b).

Cell Cultures
It has been demonstrated that cell cultures of *E. purpurea* and *E. angustifolia* can provide quantities of active echinacea compounds, including polysaccharides and phenylpropanes (cinnamic, caffeic, and ferulic acids) (Roesler *et al.*, 1991; Sícha *et al.*, 1989, 1991).

PHARMACOLOGY

Eclectic doctors learned of the potential of echinacea from the Native Americans (through Meyer) and developed the clinical use of it in this country. Homeopaths brought it to Europe (Wood, 1925) and began experimenting with it and writing about it in the 1920s and 1930s. Gerhard Madaus, founder of the pharmaceutical manufacturing firm, Madaus AG, was the first to report on his clinical and laboratory work with the genus. Auster & Schafer (1957) report that Madaus went to the U.S. for seeds of *E. angustifolia*, which was the best-known and studied species of the time, only to discover later that he was growing *E. purpurea*. This was quite fortuitous, because the former plant will not grow nearly as well in Germany as the latter—and some studies suggest that *E. purpurea* has shown stronger immune-stimulating properties than *E. angustifolia*. They are probably comparable in strength.

From this beginning and the first work in the laboratory in Germany in the 1930s, there have been over 400 journal articles published on the chemistry, pharmacology, and clinical uses of echinacea to date.

Major Pharmacological Effects of Echinacea

• **Inhibits hyaluronidase, stimulates the production of new tissue** (Büsing, 1952; Vogel & Mitarb, 1968; Bonadeo, 1971) Bonadeo and his group proposed that an uncharacterized polysaccharide they called Echinacin B forms a complex with hyaluronic acid, making it resistant to attack by hyaluronidase, which in turn leads to an increase in hyaluronic acid production, fibrosis, and the formation of fibroblasts necessary for wound healing.

- **Acts as a weak antibiotic** (Stroll, *et al.*, 1950)
A fragment of the echinacoside molecule (6.3 mg) was found to be equal in strength to 1 unit of penicillin. Schulte *et al.* (1967) isolated four bacteriostatic and fungistatic polyacetylenes from *E. purpurea* and *E. angustifolia*.

- **Has anti-inflammatory/antiphlogistic effects** (Vogel & Mitarb, 1968; Tubaro, *et al.*, 1987; Wagner *et al.*, 1989)
Echinacea extract showed antiexudative activity in rats; a polysaccharide from *E. angustifolia* showed strong anti-inflammatory activity. An alkylamide fraction from *E. purpurea* roots also displayed anti-inflammatory activity.

- **Stimulates the adrenal cortex**
Mostbeck & Studlar (1962) found that urinary corticosteroids output is increased after injections of Echinacin® (a preparation of the fresh juice of the aerial parts of *E. purpurea*), accompanied by a fall (50%) of the eosinophil count and a rise in body temperature.

- **Stimulates the properdin/complement system**
(A biochemical immune complex, which kills bacteria and viruses.) Büsing (1958) demonstrated increased properdin levels in animals after injections of Echinacin®, which were later said to be due to a stress-induced adrenocorticotropic hormone (ACTH) secretion (Büsing & Thürigen, 1959).

- **Shows interferon-like activity** (Lohmann-Matthes. 1989; Wagner, *et al.*, 1989)
The injection in animals of two high molecular weight polysaccharides from *E. purpurea* tissue cultures increased production of interferon beta$_2$ and interleukin 1 by macrophages.

- **Promotes non-specific cellular immunity** (Viehmann, 1978; Kinkel, 1984; Lasach, 1983; Vömel, 1985; Wagner, *et al.*, 1985; Wagner & Jurcic, 1991).

For a review of the testing on these important effects, see also Bauer & Wagner, 1991.

ECHINACEA AS A NON-SPECIFIC IMMUNE STIMULANT

Early Work

The plant's anti-inflammatory and antiseptic effect is reportedly due to its action supporting the opsonic index (increases phagocytosis, the process of engulfing other cells or foreign particles by phagocyte cells) and stimulation of the leukocytes (Unruh, 1915; Wood, 1925: Kuhn, 1953).

Tests with the Fresh-Pressed Juice of *Echinacea purpurea*

In vitro tests, animal experiments, and tests with human volunteers show that echinacea preparations increase the number and phagocytic activity of granulocytes, also called neutrophils, (Choné, 1969; Möse, 1983; Stotzem, *et al.*, 1992) and macrophages (Leng-Peschlow, 1992). A stimulation of granulocytes and macrophages, which have their precursors in the bone-marrow, is significant because these carry the chief load in the body's defense against bacterial and viral infections (Wagner & Jurcic, 1991).

Stuppner (1985) showed that freeze-dried EP *(Echinacea purpurea)* fresh juice clearly showed phagocytosis-raised activities in different dilutions (10^{-3} to 10^{-5} mg/ml) *in vitro*, as well as in the granulocyte and the carbon clearance test. In higher concentrations, the echinacea fresh-pressed juice was immunosuppressive and also cytotoxic.

That granulocytes and macrophages are stimulated by echinacea is also confirmed by studies that show an increase in chemotaxis, bacteria killing capacity (Krause, 1986), properdin (Reissmann, 1966), tumor necrosis factor (Fontana), and interleukin-1 (Miller). In an animal test model (carbon-clearance test), Echinacin® showed a normalizing effect on the RES (reticuloendothelial system), when certain of its functions (such as phagocytosis) were suppressed by the administration of broad-spectrum antibiotics (Bittner, 1969).

Tymper, *et al.* (1987) developed a method utilizing Echinacin® and other substances for testing the performance of phagocytosis in human granulocytes. The authors state that through the test, inborn or acquired defects of the efficiency of phagocytosis can be detected, playing a special role in the evaluation of the course of chronic diseases.

Lücker (1982) demonstrated that injections of Echinacin® (0.1 g) in humans could lead to a transitory elevation of the general leucocyte count which reached a maximum after four hours. Eight hours after the application it returned to the baseline value. Particularly, neutrophil levels were raised above those of a placebo group, eosinophil levels were diminished (even after eight hours) and lymphocyte levels fell off after 3-4 hours.

Lasch *et al.* (1983) found that injections of Echinacin® in healthy men (n=12) led to an increase of phagocytotic activity against *Candida albicans.* There was no effect on natural killer cells. In a controlled experiment with 12 healthy men, Echinacin® by intramuscular injection stimulated phagocytosis of granulocytes against *Candida albicans* (up to 50% after 3-4 days) (Möse, 1983).

A stimulation of the bone marrow (where immune effector cells arise) can be supported by the observation that in *in vitro* experiments the bone-marrow reserve is depleted and the proliferation of granuloblasts and macrophages is stimulated with administration of echinacea (Krause, 1984).

Coeugniet (1987) showed that the cell-mediated immunity was strengthened in human patients with recurrent *Candida* and Herpes simplex infections and cervical, ovarian and breast cancer when Echinacin® and thymus extract were administered.

A number of recent studies using chemotherapy (cyclophosphamide) in low doses in conjunction with Echinacin® have been reported in patients with advanced pancreatic cancer (Lersch, *et al.*, 1990a) and hepatocellular cancer (Lersch, *et al.*, 1990). The Echinacin® was responsible for counteracting some aspects of immune suppression often seen with chemotherapy, by stimulating phagocytic cells and modulating other immune parameters. The survival rate of inoperable metastasizing cancers was lengthened in some patients and the quality of life was said to be improved, due partly to the increased tolerance of the lower doses of the cyclophosphamide.

Tests with *Echinacea angustifolia, E. pallida,* and *E. purpurea*

Bauer, *et al.*, (1988d, 1989) tested aerial parts and roots of all three commercial species (EA, EP, EPA) using oral application of ethanolic extracts in mice. They found all parts stimulated phagocytosis, but *E. purpurea* showed the strongest activity. Interestingly, when the extract was too diluted, (below 10^{-7} mg ml^{-1}) it had no effect; when it was too concentrated (above 10^{-2} mg ml^{-1}), it actually suppressed phagocytosis. The active compounds were thought to include polyacetylenes, alkylamides, an essential oil, and cichoric acid; Echinacoside was inactive. The aerial parts of the three species showed less activity than the roots, and the lipophilic fraction was always more active than the hydrophilic fraction.

Jurcic, *et al.*, (1989) studied a standardized alcoholic extract of *E. purpurea* root administered orally (3 x 30 drops) to healthy men (n=12), and noted a clear increase in immune activity (granulocyte phagocytosis) over a placebo group (n=12). Maximum stimulation was seen on the 5th day (120%), declining to normal 3 days after the dose was discontinued.

Tests with the Polysaccharide Fraction

A number of tests have demonstrated stimulation of macrophages and other immune effector cells *in vivo* and *in vitro*—especially active are high molecular weight polysaccharides. This effect has also been noted for a number of other plants, including *Eleutherococcus senticosus*, so-called Siberian ginseng.

Commercial quantities of purified Echinacea polysaccharides (EP) (from cell cultures) have been extensively studied and found to very selectively stimulate macrophage activity and killing ability, enhance the activities of polymorphonuclear cells (PMN) and stimulate macrophages to increase their secretion of tumor necrosis factor (TNF-), release of interferon beta$_2$, interleukin-1 (IL-1), interleukin-6 (IL-6), and production of oxygen radicals, which greatly inhibited the growth of *Candida albicans*. Monocytes showed increased secretion of TNT-, IL-6 and IL-1, as well as increased ability to mediate the proliferation of lymphocytes (Roesler *et al.*, 1991a,b). The polysaccharide preparation also increased proliferation of phagocytes in the spleen and bone marrow as well as migration of granulocytes in the peripheral blood. B- and T-cells were not stimulated [note: B- and T- cell functions are related to the "specific" immune function, but are included in this section because of space considerations.]

In a separate test with EP, the researchers were able to demonstrate some of the same increases in immune function, and in addition, a slight stimulation in the proliferation of T-cells (Luettig, 1989).

The polysaccharides have been tested mainly by injection (in animals and humans), and it is still controversial as to whether they act orally, but Bauer & Wagner (1991) have concluded that "polysaccharides may be implicated in the activity of expressed Echinacea juice (Echinacin®) and aqueous extracts and in the response to the oral administration of powdered whole drug." One of the most common arguments against EP having an immuno-stimulating effect orally is the proposal that such large molecules will break down when they encounter the hydrochloric acid in the stomach, reducing or eliminating their effectiveness. However, it is already known that such high-molecular weight cell-wall molecules are not affected by stomach acid (Hentges, 1983). Although Bauer and others have stated that these polysaccharides do not survive in high-alcohol (ethanolic) tinctures, Echinacin® itself contains about 22% ethanol; the manufacturer has stated that the main active constituents of this preparation are the high-molecular weight polysaccharides.

Homeopathic Preparations

Möller & Naumann (1987) administered intramuscular injections of a homeopathic Echinacea preparation (D4) (once daily for 3 days) to a group of patients with low leukocyte counts due to viral infection and saw a 27% increase in leukocyte levels. Rapid improvements in the conditions of the patients were seen.

Note: Most, but not all of the research quoted above was performed with a fresh *E. purpurea* juice preparation, Echinacin®, but for these effects to be fully credible regarding the clinical application, further human studies are needed (Schiedges, 1992).

Effects on the "Specific" Immune Functions (T-cells)

In patients with acute inflammation associated with viral (n=9) and bacterial (n=14) infections, a decrease in T-helper (T-4) cells and no change in T-suppressor (T-8) cells after injection of Echinacin® for 7 days, 2 ml twice daily, with a corresponding overall increase in lymphocyte count was noted (Gaisbauer *et al.*, 1986). A similar study reported by Gaisbauer showed virtually the same results (Gaisbauer, 1990a).

Coeugniet & Elek (1987) saw a slight transitory decrease in T-4 cells (ca. 3%) in patients with contact eczema (n=4), neurodermatitis (n=6), *Herpes simplex* (n=8) and *Candida albicans* infection (n=10), 24 hours after a single injection of Echinacin®, with a gradual 14% rise in T-cells (maximum after 8 days), with T-8 levels essentially remaining the same. When a single injection was given daily, the T-4 levels remained low, but increased after a week with no injections. The authors emphasize that "daily therapy = inhibition" (of the cell-mediated immunity) and "intermittent therapy = stimulation." They say that continuous therapy may be useful for an overactive cell-mediated immunity (allergies, autoimmune disorders), whereas intermittent therapy may be useful for the "therapy of cell-mediated immune deficiency."

All studies in this section were performed with injections of Echinacin®; there is presently no data for the influence of echinacea products on T-4 levels with oral application.

Anti-Viral Activity

The juice of the fresh tops of *E. purpurea* enhanced the anti-viral activity (against herpes and influenza) of mouse cell cultures, especially when pretreated 4-6 hours before exposure (Wacker & Hilbig, 1978). In an antiviral screening study, May & Willuhn (1978) found that an *E. purpurea* (perhaps the adulterant *Parthenium integrifolium?*) root water extract (1:10) inhibited the herpes and influenza virus in vitro, but not the polio virus. An *E. angustifolia* (possibly *E. pallida?*) root extract showed no activity. Eilmes (1976) demonstrated a viral-protective effect on cultured cells with both aqueous and methanol extracts of *E. angustifolia* roots. Combining both extracts led to a stronger activity.

Local (Topical) Applications

Echinacea preparations are often used in Europe, and increasingly in the U.S. and other countries, for topical application for wound-healing (see Clinical section). This use is supported by *in vitro* and *in vivo* tests that show echinacea can activate the non-specific cellular immune system by direct contact of cells and tissues (as opposed to stimulation via i.v., i.p., or oral application) (Kuhn, 1953). More specifically, tests have shown that there is an increased occurrence of histiogenic phagocytes (histiocytes, which are a type of mononuclear phagocyte tending to concentrate in the connective tissue), increased occurrence of hemotogenic phagocytes (granulocytes) in tissue accompanied by increased phagocytosis, chemotaxis and bactericide capacity, and activation and proliferation of fibrocytes and fibroblasts (leading to increased production of hyaluronic acid and other constituents of the intercellular cement, which act as a barrier toward pathogens (Koch, 1953), as well as the often-quoted anti-hyaluronidase activity (Koch, 1952).

A Laboratory Study Showing No Activity

Interestingly, in one study, researchers (Schumacher & Friedberg, 1991) could detect no immune stimulation (using the carbon-clearance model) with either a water-soluble plant extract of *E.*

angustifolia, echinacoside, and several patent remedies containing echinacea. The extracts were applied to mice i.p., i.v., and orally for up to 28 days. Perhaps this study emphasizes the possible sensitive dose-dependent nature of echinacea preparations, as Coeugniet and Elek (1987) also mention. Bauer has stated that a potential problem with some studies is the failure to properly identify the plant material extract. In the above study, a high-alcohol non-standardized tincture (60% ethanol) of *E. angustifolia* (possibly *E. pallida?*) was used, which probably contained no immune-stimulating polysaccharides. After the alcohol was removed, the aqueous solution was freeze-dried and then dissolved in water, which would eliminate any lipophilic alkylamides (also known to be immune stimulating). Thus, the preparation used in the study may not have contained either of the two main fractions known to be immuno-active (Bauer, 1993).

MODERN CLINICAL WORK

With all the interest in echinacea and its commercial preparations, it is interesting that there have been only a few controlled double-blind clinical trials to verify the cultural and medical uses.

However, there have been numerous clinical reports about the use of echinacea, nearly all with the fresh stabilized *E. purpurea* juice, Echinacin®, in the injectible form, although a few have been conducted with oral applications or an externally applied salve. As interesting and suggestive as these studies are, they are not indicative of clinical application outside of Europe (especially the U.S., Canada, New Zealand, and Australia where oral echinacea preparations are popular), where echinacea in this form is rarely, if ever used. A few other studies have been performed with combination products such as Esberitox®, which, besides echinacea, contains extracts of *Baptisia tinctoria* (Wild indigo) and *Thuja occidentalis* (Arbor vitae). There are over 200 studies to report here, so only representative citations will be given in Table 10. In nearly every case, a favorable outcome was reported with the echinacea treatment. Many of these trials are uncontrolled and would not stand up to today's strict standards for clinical testing; however, they do have merit in representing actual clinical experience with the preparation. For a comprehensive review, see Hobbs (1989) and Foster (1991).

Table 10
Clinical Reports with Commercial Echinacea Products

In injectible form (Echinacin®, unless otherwise noted):

- General infection and wound healing (Sickel, 1971; Quadripur, 1976a,b)
- Polyarthritis (Meixner, 1953; Reuss, 1986)
- Influenza and colds (Hunsdorfer, 1954; Hansen, 1965)
- Pertussis in children (Baetgen, 1984; Volz, 1957; Zimmermann, 1969)
- Disturbed sleep in children with pertussis (Sprockhoff, 1986)
- Upper respiratory tract infections, chronic in children (Tympner, 1978)
- Tuberculosis (Heesen, 1964)
- Bronchitis (Baetgen, 1988; Sprockhoff, 1964)
- Tonsillitis, otitis media in pediatrics (Sprockhoff, 1964)
- Eczema (Tronnier, 1967)
- Psoriasis (Korting and Rasp, 1954; Brehm, 1962; [oral] Gaertner, 1963)
- Warts (Franken and Sönnichsen, 1966)
- Chronic Prostatitis (Herrmann, 1952; Bauer, 1958)
- Urogenital infections (Uhlmann, 1958; Weissbach, *et al.*, 1977)
- Allergies (Reith, 1978)
- Candidiasis (Lasch, *et al.*, 1983; Coeugniet and Kühnast, 1986)
- Gynecological infections (Höreth and Heiss, 1957; Tosetti, K., 1961)
- Pelvic inflammatory disease (P.I.D.) (Röseler, 1952; Schuster, 1952)
- Chronic osteomyelitis (Hanfstaengel, 1956)
- Pancreatic, esophageal, colorectal cancer (Lersch, *et al.*, 1992), hepatocellular cancer (Lersch, *et al.*, 1990)(with chemotherapy)
- Chronic skin ulcers (Bohl, 1954)
- Frostbite and gunshot wounds (Giesbert, 1943)

Topical Use of Echinacea Preparations (Echinacin® ointment)

- A 5-month trial (not controlled) with 4,598 patients and 538 doctors concerning the healing of inflammatory skin conditions, wounds, eczema, burns, *Herpes simplex* and varicose ulceration of the leg. Overall, a favorable result was seen in 85.5% of the patients (Viehmann, 1978).
- A report on 38 years of clinical experience with the ointment in general practice for healing a variety of skin conditions showed good results (Sickel, 1971).
- Good results with ulcerative gingivitis and mixed parodontopathy (Gasiorowska, 1981).

Table 10 (Continued)

Clinical Trials with Oral Application of Echinacin® Liquid and other Echinacea Preparations

- Psoriasis (Gärtner, 1963)
- Candidiasis, recurrent—good effect (with a reduction in recurrent infections) with oral Echinacin® (Coeugniet & Kühnast, 1986)
- Upper respiratory tract infections

In a double-blind, placebo-controlled study with 180 volunteers (Bräunig, et al., 1992), it was determined that 2 droppersful of an *Echinacea purpurea* (herb) unstandardized alcoholic extract (1:5, 55% ethanol) were only as effective as a placebo preparation (55% ethanol, 45% water, sugar coloring) in relieving symptoms of, and duration of, flu-like infections; whereas the improvement with 4 droppersful compared to placebo was statistically significant. An effect from the higher dose was seen after 3-4 days, but the full effect was not seen until 8-10 days.

In another double-blind, placebo-controlled study with 108 human volunteers who had chronic upper respiratory tract infections (more than 3 occurrences of such infections as otitis, ear canal catarrh, rhinitis, tonsillitis, pharyngitis, laryngitis, bronchitis, pneumonia, sinusitis, etc., in a half year), Echinacin® (2 x 4 ml/day) was given over an 8-week period. Compared to the placebo group, in the echinacea group, "36% more patients suffered no infections," the time between infections was lengthened, the duration of illness was shortened, and severity of symptoms was lessened. The echinacea preparation was well-tolerated, and patients with lowered T4/T8 ratios seemed to profit most from the treatment (Schöneberger, 1992).

- General immune stimulation

A few tests on humans have shown Echinacea to exhibit clinically significant activation of macrophage and granulocyte activity, with an increase of phagocytosis (Jurcic, et al., 1989).

Clinical Trials With Oral Application of Esberitox® and Other Compound Preparations Containing Echinacea

- Lowered white blood cell count after radiation therapy for cancer (Pohl, 1969; Sartor, 1972)
- Influenza and colds (Kleinschmidt, 1965; Freyer, 1974; Ammann and Suter, 1987)
- Urogenital infection (Felder, 1959)
- Two placebo-controlled, double-blind studies, with 100 flu patients each, showed a significant shortening of the duration of the flu and a reduction of the severity of the symptoms (Vorberg and Schneider, 1989; Dorn, 1989).
- As a prophylactic in a double-blind study, with 650 students, a clear reduction in the frequency of infection was shown, especially statistically significant in persons with a heightened tendency towards infection (Schmidt, et al., 1990).

TOXICOLOGY

Historical human use and experimental animal studies indicate little need for concern regarding the safety of echinacea.

Lang and Mengs (1976a,b) found no toxic symptoms in mice and rats given Echinacin® i.v. The LD50 (dose at which 50% of the animals died) for both animals was determined to be 1.25 g, representing 50 ml of Echinacin®/kg i.v. Subsequently, Mengs (1985), in an unpublished study, reported that Echinacin® was "well tolerated" by both animals, and caused no adverse effects after successive doses higher than 8.0 ml/kg (a very high dose).

In 1985, two studies were performed by Microtest Research Ltd. in York, England (Kennelly, 1985a; Kennelly, 1985b). In the first controlled study, Echinacin® showed no mutagenic activity in four strains of *Salmonella typimurium*, when tested up to a concentration of 5000 ug/plate, under these assay conditions either in the absence or presence of metabolic activation. The second study showed that Echinacin® was not able to induce significant levels of micronuclei in the bone marrow cells of mice treated with the acute oral toxicity limit dose of 2 g/kg.

Lenk (1989) showed that several Echinacea polysaccharides, first isolated by Wagner, *et al.*, have very low acute toxicity. He determined the LD50 of polysaccharide-rich fractions from *E. purpurea* to be between 1000 and 2500 mg/kg in the mice.

Schimmer *et al.*, (1989) were able to show that a neutral immuno-active polysaccharide from *E. purpurea* cell cultures (NFA 10) had no mutagenic activity *in vitro* in cultures of human lymphocytes, even with repeated, long-term testing.

Mengs, *et al.*, (1991) administered doses of an expressed juice of *E. purpurea* tops to rats, both orally (up to 8000 mg/kg/day) and i.v. many times the human therapeutic dose and could find no toxic effects. The group also tested the extract for mutagenicity with microorganisms and mammalian cells *in vitro* and in mice with negative results. They concluded that the juice was "virtually non-toxic."

For more complete reviews see Schimmel and Werner, 1981 (Echinacin®); Bauer and Wagner, 1990, 1991; Hobbs, 1989; Foster, 1991.

PHARMACY AND PHARMACOGNOSY

Commercial Preparations

As immunomodulators, the popularity of echinacea preparations is increasing worldwide. For instance, in Germany (1989), the most popular echinacea product is 131st on a list of the 2,000 most-prescribed drugs (Schumacher & Friedberg, 1991), and is possibly the most popular herb in the U.S, with sales increasing dramatically over the last few years. It is obvious to the herbal consumer that there is an increasing array of echinacea products available in the natural food store or herb shop. The use of echinacea seems to "cross over" into groups of people who wouldn't normally use herbal products, and even Hollywood has discovered echinacea. It was recently reported in the popular press that celebrities such as Cher, Jodie Foster, and members of the Star Trek cast commonly use the herb to ward off colds and flu (Garstang, 1993). Much of this popularity seems to be due to simple word-of-mouth transmission.

At present, the most popular echinacea products are liquid extracts (made with varying proportions of grain alcohol and water, and, in some cases, glycerin), spray- or freeze-dried extracts in capsules and tablets, simple herb powders in capsules and tablets, and the fresh juice of *E. purpurea* tops stabilized with ethanol.

Of the proven immuno-active compounds from *Echinacea* spp., the polyacetylenes and cichoric acid are unstable and may not occur in commercial products (Bauer and Wagner, 1991, Bauer, 1991). Only the polysaccharides (though not in high-alcohol extracts) and the alkylamides are currently accepted as active in commercial products.

Common Opinions for Quality Echinacea Products
(according to leading herbalists and herbal manufacturers)

- The form (powder, liquid, etc.) is less important than the quality of the starting herb and the care taken in the manufacturing process, though most, if not all, of the clinical and laboratory tests and reports used a liquid alcoholic preparation.
- Entirely from certified organically grown plants (for the purpose of preserving wild populations, some of which are becoming endangered).
- The fresher the better. Extracts should ideally be made from the fresh plants.

- Products should contain at least one part of or a combination of the roots, leaves, and flowers of *E. purpurea* or this plus the roots of *E. angustifolia*.
- Products should be certified to contain only *Echinacea purpurea* or *E. angustifolia* (not the common adulterant *Parthenium integrifolium* or other species of *Echinacea*).
- If the product contains *E. pallida* (wild or cultivated) or *E. tennesseensis* (cultivated only!), this will be clearly noted.
- If the herb is extracted, the ideal menstruum is an ethanol to water mixture of 55/45% for the dried root (Wagner, personal communication, 1989), or about 75% for fresh roots or tops.
- Fresh juice preparations should be made from high-quality fresh plant material and properly stabilized with about 20-25% ethanol.
- Dried, powdered extracts should ideally be made from fresh material.

Some researchers have suggested that combination preparations containing more than one immuno-stimulating plant extract, such as *Baptisia tinctoria* and *Thuja occidentalis*, may be more effective than echinacea alone because of a synergistic effect, but this has yet to be proven in direct comparative human studies (Wagner and Jurcic, 1991; Schranner, *et al.*, 1989).

In Europe, a number of products derived from cell cultures of Echinacea species are being developed and tested. These cultures may have future importance in the production of large quantities of standardized "phyto-medicines" for use by physicians and some herbalists (Sícha, *et al.*, 1989).

Dosage and Duration of Application

According to Wagner and Jurcic, immune reactions work by the law of all or nothing; that is, when immune modulators (such as Echinacea products) reach a critical dose, they lead to an immune response, which cannot be further increased by raising the concentration, and may even, in some cases, lead to immune suppression (Wagner and Jurcic, 1991).

Because preliminary tests have shown the activity of echinacea extracts to be dose-dependent, there has been a call to increase the quantity and quality of testing to determine the correct dose of echinacea for effective immune-stimulation (Gaisbauer, 1990b). This may be partly answered by the placebo-controlled, double-blind study (Bräunig, *et al.*) published in 1992, previously mentioned, which showed that 180 drops of an ethanolic extract of E. *purpurea* (roots) significantly reduced the severity and duration of the symptoms of flu-like infections, whereas 90 drops was no more effective than a placebo preparation (containing ethanol and sugar coloring).

In another study (Jurcic, *et al.*, 1989), maximum immune stimulation was reached after 5 days, after which the immune stimulation began to subside, even though the preparation was continued at the same dosage.

Echinacea—Stimulant or Tonic?

At the present time, the view that Echinacea is an immune stimulant, rather than a tonic is still not without its critics. Some herbalists are of the opinion that Echinacea can be taken long-term in significant doses, and it may just keep getting better. My own experience strongly suggests that echinacea is more of a stimulant to be taken like most herbal stimulants—for short periods of time only when needed. The following discussion is offered in support of this view.

One of the strongest clinical studies showing that echinacea may lead to immune suppression if used to excess is a 1989 German study (Jurcic et al., 1989). This paper and at least one leading researcher (Dr. Rudi Bauer) involved with the study do offer support of the position that echinacea is an immune stimulant (rather than a tonic) that should be taken in cycles with short rests in between.

The following is my translation of the relevant part of this study:

"The single-blind study performed with 27 healthy volunteers (14 in the 'echinacea' group and 13 in the placebo group) showed a clear increase in phagocytosis after the first injection. This led to a maximum stimulation of about 20% after the 3rd injection of the 4th day. A difference from the placebo group was still clearly recognizable 3 days after the completion of the 5th day of treatment (when the injections were stopped). A continuous decline to the normal range resulted after 11 days. The observation that a clear decrease in activity started already after the next to last injection (as can be seen on Fig. 1 of the original article, c.h.) could mean that after a short stimulation period a fatigue or exhaustion phase can occur. Possibly the rapid decrease in activity is due to an immunosuppressive effect as a consequence of over-stimulation."

A second study was also performed with an orally-administered echinacea preparation, and a similar pattern of decline in activity was seen (the drop-off is not as dramatic as with the injections, but it is evident), but no specific discussion about immune-suppression was given.

I also asked Dr. Rudi Bauer to comment on this aspect of the study. He contends that the results of these studies have to be

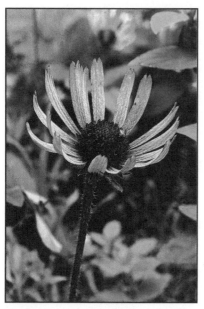

Fig. 10. *Echinacea tennesseensis*
Copyright ©1992 Steven Foster

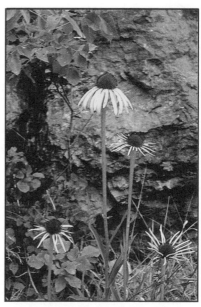

Fig. 11. *Echinacea paradoxa*
Copyright ©1992 Steven Foster

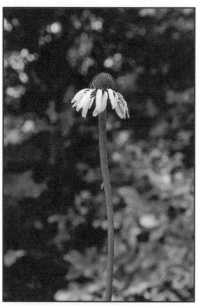

Fig. 12. *Echinacea atrorubens*
Copyright ©1992 Steven Foster

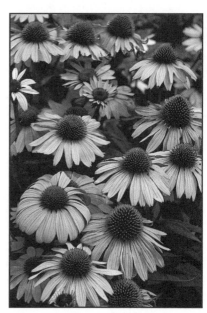

Fig. 13. *Echinacea purpurea*
Copyright ©1992 Steven Foster

Echinacea

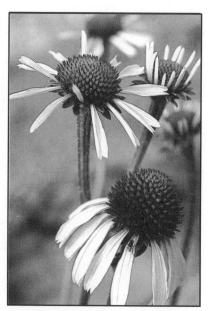

Fig. 15. *Echinacea angustifolia*
Copyright ©1992 Steven Foster

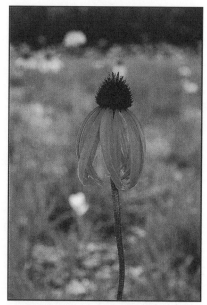

Fig. 15. *Echinacea simulata*
Copyright ©1992 Steven Foster

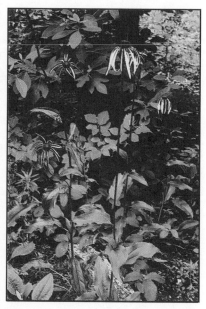

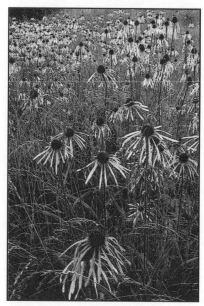

Fig. 17. *Echinacea pallida*
Copyright ©1992 Steven Foster

Fig. 16. *Echinacea laevigata*
Copyright ©1992 Steven Foster

interpreted carefully based on statistical significance—that it may be difficult to make a case (about a rapid immune suppressive effect); nevertheless,

"...there is some experience that the immune system cannot be stimulated in an unlimited form. Practical experience shows that it is best to do an interval therapy, like you have suggested. However, there are few clinical data which prove that procedure."

Another study supports the idea that intermittent use of echinacea may be more effective for immune stimulation than continuous use (Hobbs, 1994):

Coeugniet & Elek (1987) saw a slight transitory decrease in T-4 cells (ca. 3%) in patients with contact eczema (n=4), neurodermatitis (n=6), *Herpes simplex* (n=8), and *Candida albicans* infection (n=10), 24 hours after a single injection of Echinacin®, with a gradual 14% rise in T-4 cells (maximum after 8 days), with T-8 levels essentially remaining the same. When a single injection was given daily, the T-4 levels remained low, but increased after a week with no injections. The authors emphasize that "daily therapy=inhibition" (of the cell-mediated immunity), and "intermittent therapy=stimulation." They say that continuous therapy may be useful for an overactive cell-mediated immunity (allergies, autoimmune disorders), whereas intermittent therapy may be useful for the "therapy of cell-mediated immune deficiency.

Though it could certainly be argued that oral doses of echinacea are less problematic in regards to immune suppression than when administered by injection, there are reports that oral echinacea has a very similar effect in the way in which it affects the immune system (Coeugniet and Kühanast, 1986).

In fact, this study seems to contradict my above contentions by showing a cellular immune activity increase (in the oral group) over a period of 10 weeks, as well as fewer recurrences of chronic candidiasis in a group of 203 patients. However, this study proves nothing either way, because the study did not include a control group with placebo to compensate for the immune-strengthening effects of simply receiving the echinacea preparation, as well as being a part of the "Echinacin® group", accompanied by extra attention from the researchers, etc. It is well-known that the placebo effect can elicit a significant immune response from individuals (Kelkar and Ross, 1994).

There are two parts to this discussion. First, is echinacea a stimulant which, according to Traditional Chinese Medicine, should be taken for a short period of time to reduce heat or help rid the body of a pathogenic influence, and then be discontinued, or can it be given steadily in any amount desired (similar to a food) to help support and nourish the body? My experience, as well as a good knowledge of the scientific literature available, points strongly to the former idea. I have observed these limitations in echinacea therapy from personal experience over 10 years of extensive use. To me, it only makes sense that the body's immune system will accommodate to such stimulation over a period of time—and can become actually suppressed if too high a dose is given for a specific individual. Second, if we accept that echinacea is a stimulant, what are the optimum periods for dose vs. rest periods? My experience is that this depends on the type of echinacea preparation (whether high- or low-alcohol preparation, part of plant used, which species), the individual's constitutional make-up and diet (etc.), the clinical setting, and perhaps other unknown factors. My opinion is that the optimum time period is anywhere between 10 days and a month, but usually about 10-14 days, with a rest period between dose periods. If several cycles of echinacea treatment do not seem to help produce a reduction in the signs of an infection, then it is time to examine the person's constitution more closely—often the strategy then is to build up the yin (perhaps adrenal cortex insufficiency) because the heat of infection is "false heat," instead of trying to rouse a tired horse (the immune system and adrenal-pituitary axis).

In conclusion, the jury is still out about these issues, but I feel the evidence and experience is strong enough to recommend to practitioners and consumers of echinacea products to use a cyclic dose pattern and not to continue large doses (over 2-3 droppersful of the liquid extract) for extended periods.

Adulterants

Echinacea is a plant remedy that has been commonly adulterated in the market throughout its commercial history. The most common adulterant now is *Parthenium integrifolium*, which is often sold as *E. purpurea*.

It has become evident through the work of Steven Foster (1985a, b), Rudolf Bauer (1987c), and others, that most of the commercially available root of *Echinacea purpurea* on the U. S. market was (before about 1988) in fact, *Parthenium*. Fortunately, many commercial product manufacturers have switched to certified organic herb in the last few years. Fresh *E. purpurea* products from above ground parts have not been affected by adulteration.

In 1987, a number of American manufacturers met under the auspices of the American Herbal Products Association (AHPA) and agreed to not sell *Parthenium* as Echinacea and to make *Parthenium* products labeled as such.

This adulteration is not new. Herb sellers have been substituting *Parthenium*, especially for *E. purpurea,* for well over 80 years, probably because the roots of *Parthenium* are much weightier and easier to harvest, and because populations of wild *E. purpurea* are scattered and sparse. In all likelihood, any commercial root products or bulk herb of *E. purpurea* that did not originate from a *cultivated* source are probably *Parthenium integrifolium* (Foster, 1990). John Uri Lloyd noted a "spurious adulterant" later identified as *P. integrifolium* in 1910 (J. Moser 1910).

Besides *Parthenium, E. pallida* is also sold as *E. angustifolia* (Bauer, 1991b), and this is rarely mentioned on product labels and in accompanying literature (author's observation). While this latter species may have immune-activating properties, and it was formerly official in the *National Formulary*, it has not undergone the extensive testing that the other two species have, and therefore should be clearly marked when it is included in commercial products.

Other plants that were formerly substituted for commercial *Echinacea* sp. include *Lespedeza capitata* (bush clover) and *Eryngium aquaticum* (eryngo) (Lloyd, 1917).

Analysis of the Crude Herb and Commercial Products

Analysis of commercial supplies and products of echinacea is by visual inspection, taste, microscopic analysis, and chemical analysis by thin-layer chromatography (TLC) or high-performance liquid chromatography (HPLC). It has recently become obvious, through increased scrutiny and regulatory pressures, that insuring the proper identity and even quality of commercial supplies of echinacea (and other herbs as well) is essential if the herb industry is to continue to mature.

The following analytical methods can be consulted for identification/differentiation of the species. See also Bauer and Wagner (1990, 1991).

- Microscopic, botanical analysis: Kraemer and Sollenberger, 1911; Heubl, *et al.*, 1988; Heubl and Bauer, 1990; Schulthess, *et al.*, 1991 (achenes).
- TLC analysis: Bauer, *et al.*, 1986, 1987
- HPLC analysis: Bauer, *et al.*, 1987; Bauer *et al.*, 1988e; Schulthess, *et al.*, 1991 (identification and differentiation of the 3 main commercial species from the achenes).

STANDARDIZATION

Although some European products use echinacoside as a reference standard (author's observation), a study published in 1991 (Schumacher & Friedberg) has supported the previously held finding that this compound is not particularly active; also, it is not present in *E. purpurea*. Other active compounds, such as alkylamides, may be the best candidates for eventual standardization. Recently, a super-critical CO_2 extract of *E. purpurea* root said to contain about 50% alkylamides was claimed in a Japanese patent to be useful for inflammation, edema, and immune disorders (Etsuio and Enriko, 1992; Schulthess, *et al.*, 1991).

Wagner and Jurcic (1991) reported that the concentration for active low-molecular weight compounds is often in the range of 0.1 to 1%. High molecular-weight compounds (such as polysaccharides or glycoproteins) are difficult to isolate and characterize, but Esberitox® is now standardized to glycoproteins, and commercial products standardized to polysaccharides from cell cultures are under development.

CULTIVATION

Because of the rapidly dwindling supplies of wild plants, the commercial organic cultivation of echinacea is of extreme importance. It has been reported that over 100,000 pounds of wild echinacea have been harvested and shipped overseas for many years, and demand in the U.S. has dramatically increased since the mid-1980s. As the popularity of echinacea has increased over the last 10 years, the wild supplies are increasingly pressured, leading to over-harvesting and the harvesting of endangered or rare species. High-quality wild-crafted *E. angustifolia* has been increasingly difficult to find in the 1991-1993 seasons.

Fortunately, there are at least two large suppliers of certified-organically grown *E. purpurea*, and to a lesser extent, *E. angustifolia* and *E. pallida*, though the latter plant is not as commercially popular as the first two. Based on projections for future demand, focus on echinacea cultivation by organic growers would seem commercially feasible (Blumenthal, 1993).

Specific cultivation techniques will not be included here, but thorough reviews are available (Hobbs, 1989; Foster, 1991).

Appendix 2
Summary of Indications and Doses

The following is a partial list of ailments where
Echinacea may be of value.

1. Any infection, chronic or acute, but especially where there is not long-term immune deficiency or dysfunction. Echinacea is also used (especially in Europe) as an adjuvant therapy with antibiotics and chemotherapy. For serious ailments or emergency conditions, echinacea is best used as an adjuvant therapy to support other treatments.

- *Colds or influenza*, especially before onset, or in early stages.
- *Candidiasis*
- *Strep throat*, as a gargle, solution swallowed.
- *Staph. infections*, impetigo, under nails, etc.
- *Urinary tract infections*, cystitis, urethritis especially.
- *Pelvic Inflammatory Disease* (P.I.D.)
- *Tonsil and throat infections*, as a gargle, solution swallowed.
- *Infected wounds* that are hard to heal.
- *Burns*, topically and internally.
- *Herpes*, topically and internally.
- *Skin ulcers*, keep the area moist with Echinacea extract.
- *Eczema*
- *Psoriasis*, taken internally and applied externally.
- *Whooping cough*
- *Bronchitis*

2. For *leucopenia* (low leucocyte count) due to radiation therapy or other causes, when not directly related to long-term deficiency of immune function and cellular nutrition, protein-carbohydrate deficiency, malabsorption, or abusive life-style.

3. *Rheumatoid arthritis*, for its anti-inflammatory effect.

4. As an *anti-allergy treatment* for food allergy, environmental sensitivity and hay fever, when not related to general, long-term immune deficiency.

5. For *toothache, mouth and gum infections,* gargle, apply undiluted liquid extract directly to affected area, swish with diluted extract, and take internally.

6. *Bites* of all kinds: insect bites and stings, animal bites including rattlesnake bites (in addition to other emergency medical treatment). Applied full-strength on the bite, taken internally.

7. *Blood poisoning, food poisoning.* Large doses internally (40 drops or 4 capsules every two hours).

8. *Boils, carbuncle, abscesses,* applied externally, taken internally.

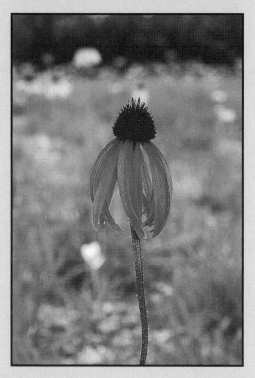

Fig. 18
Echinacea simulata

NOTES

• For *external* application, Echinacea salve or ointment is used. The liquid extract applied on a cotton pad and fixed in place, or a tea of the root or leaves is made and applied. In infections, the dressing is changed often and more Echinacea applied.

• For *internal* use, use as a *tonic* to the "surface" secretory immune function (through the macrophages) for protection against infections; 10-25 drops per day of the liquid, or 1-2 capsules or tablets (author's experience).

• For *acute infection*, a full dose is 50 drops (about one dropperful) or 300-400 mg of a dry extract 3 times daily (Wagner and Jurcic, 1991)—(or more).

• Doses between the above extremes can be taken, depending on personal needs, body weight, state of health and illness.

Appendix 3
Definition of Immunological Terms

The main effector cells of the immune system include:

Granulocytes (a group of immune cells that have granules in their cytoplasm, of 3 types:)

1) Basophils: (less than 1% of total) non-phagocytic cells that produce chemicals such as histamine; may play a role in allergic and anaphylaxis reactions

2) Eosinophils: (1-4% of total) phagocytic potential (ingests antigen-antibody complexes), plays an important role in anaphylactic and allergic reactions.

3) Neutrophils: (50-70% of total) a killer cell (by phagocytosis) which plays a major role in protecting the host against infections.

Leukocytes: the white blood cells, comprising all immune cells mentioned here.

Lymphocytes: a group of cells involved in cell-mediated immunity (such as the T-helper and T-suppressor cells) and humoral immunity (such as the B-cells that produce antibodies) that play a major role in "specific defenses" against foreign invaders. In other words, they recognize particular chemical markers on virus-infected cells and bacteria (among others) and target their bearers for destruction.

Macrophages: arising from monocytes, these "big eaters" are large, major phagocytic cells which destroy foreign invaders, toxic chemicals, and tumor cells, among other things.

Opsonic Index: a measure of the ability of the immune system to destroy pathogens by phagocytosis after they are acted on by the antibody opsonin.

Phagocyte: any number of immune cells that act to destroy bacteria and other pathogens, cellular debris, and chemicals by ingesting them (e.g. macrophages).

RES: the reticuloendothelial system: centered in the reticular connective tissue of the spleen, liver, and lymphoid tissues, it is a mononuclear phagocytic system.

References for Part I

1. Lyons, A.B. 1907. *Plant Names Scientific and Popular.* Detroit: Nelson, Baker & Co.
2. Hobbs, C. 1989. *The Echinacea Handbook.* Portland: Eclectic Medical Publications. Call Botanica Press for order form: (408) 464-7142
3. Gilmore, A. 1911. Uses of Plants by the Indians of the Missouri River Region. *Bur. Amer. Eth. Ann. Rep.* 33: 368.
4. Bauer, R. 1989. Personal communication.
5. Lloyd, J.U. 1917. *A Treatise on Echinacea.* Cincinnati: Lloyd Bros. Reprinted by Herb Pharm, Williams, OR.
6. Ellingwood, F. 1898. *American Materia Medica, Therapeutics and Pharmacognosy.* Chicago: Chicago Medical Press. Reprinted by Eclectic Medical Publications, Portland, 1983.
7. Bauer, R. and H. Wagner. 1988. "Echinacea—Der Sonnenhut—Stand der Forschung." *Zeit Phytother* 9: 151.
8. Kleinschmidt, H. 1965. Study on reduction of infection in infants with Esberitox. *Ther. d Gegen.* 1258.
9. Helbig, G. 1961. Non-specific immune-therapy in infection prophylaxis. *Med. Klin.* 56: 1512.
10. Freyer, H.U. 1974. Frequency of common infection in childhood and likelihood of prophylaxis. *Forschrift der Ther.* 92: 165.
11. Amman, M. & K. Suter. 1987. Echinacea combination: effectiveness and compatibility in cases of flu and inflammation of the nose and pharynx. *Deut. Apoth.-Zeit.* 127: 853.
12. Bauer, R., et al. 1988a. Immunological *in vivo* and *in vitro* examinations of Echinacea extracts. *Arzn.-Forsch.* 38: 276.
13. Bauer, R. 1989. Influence of Echinacea extracts on phagocytotic activity. *Zeit. Phytother.* 10: 43.
14. Lohmann-Matthes, M. L. & H. Wagner. 1989. Macrophage activation by plant polysaccharides. *Zeit. Phytother.* 10: 52.
15. Bauer, R. 1989, op cit.
16. Lasch, H.G. 1983. The effect of Echinacin on phagocytosis and natural killer cells. *Die Med. Welt.* 34: 1463.
17. Wagner, H. & A. Proksch. 1985. *Economic and Medicinal Plant Research,* vol. 1. Orlando: Academic Press, p. 113.
18. Enbergs, H. & A. Woestmann. 1986. The effect of Echinacea angustifolia on phagocytic activity of peripheral leukocytes of rabbits. *Tierärztliche Umschau* 11: 878.
19. Coeugniet, E. & R. Kühnast. 1986. Recurrent candidiasis: adjuvant immunotherapy with different formulations of echinacin." *Therapiewoche* 36: 3352.
20. Bensky, D. & A. Gamble. 1986. *Chinese Herbal Medicine, Materia Medica.* Seattle: Eastland Press.
21. Bullock, C. 1984. Two Chinese herbs show blooming anticancer potential. *Texas Med. Trib.*
22. Wenbin, C., et al. 1983. *J. Trad. Chin. Med.* 3: 63.
23. James, J. 1986. AIDS *Treatment News* 19.
24. Chone, B. & G. Manidakis. 1969. Echinacin-test on leukocyte production in radiation therapy. *Deut. Med. Woch.* 27: 1406.
25. Guan, H.C. & Z. Cong. 1982. *Yaoxue Tongbao* 17: 177.
26. Hobbs, C. R. 1985. *Usnea and other medicinal lichens: the herbal antibiotics.* Box 742, Capitola, CA: Botanica Press.

27. Hobbs, C. 1989. Feverfew. *HerbalGram* 20: 26-36. (to order subscription or back issues: 1-800-373-7105)
28. Wagner, et al. 1988. Immunologische In-vitro-und In-vivo-Untersuchungen von Arzneiprä paraten. *Phytotherapie.* Stuttgart: Hippokrates Verlag, pp. 127-135.
29. Jurcic, K., et al. 1989. Two test-subject studies for the stimulation of granulocyte phagocytosis by Echinacea-containing preparations. *Zeit. Phytother.* 10 (2): 67-70.
30. Hobbs, *The Echinacea Handbook, op cit.*
31. Geller, C.A. 1988. Personal Communication.
32. McGregor, R.L. 1968. The Taxonomy of the Genus Echinacea (Compositae). *Univ. of Kansas Sci. Bul.* 48: 132.
33. Bauer, R. & P. Remiger. 1989. TLC and HPLC analysis of alkamides in *Echinacea* drugs. *Planta Med.* 55: 367-78.
34. Foster, S. 1986. *Echinacea Exalted,* 2nd rev. ed. Brixey, MO: Ozark Beneficial Plant Project.
35. Moring, S. & C. Hobbs. 1988. Unpublished results.
36. McGregor, *op cit.*
37. Bauer, R. 1987. Personal communication.
38. King, C.J. 1971. *Freeze-drying of foods.* Cleveland, OH: CRC Press.
39. Goldblift, F.A., ed. *Freeze-drying and advanced food technology.* New York: Academic Press.

References for Appendix I

Ammann, M. and K. Suter. 1987. *Deut. Apoth. Zeit.* 127: 853.

Auster, F. and J. Schafer. 1957. *Echinacea angustifolia.* VEB G. Thieme, Leipzig.

Baetgen, D. 1984. *Therapiewoche* 34: 5115.

Baetgen, D. 1988. *T.W. Pädiatrie* 1: 66.

Bauer, K. M. 1958. *Landarzt* 34: 5115-9.

Bauer, R. and H. Wagner. 1990. *Echinacea, Wissenshaftliche.* Stuttgart: Verlagsgesellschaft.

Bauer, R., P. Remiger, and E. Alstat. 1990b. *Planta Med.* 56: 533-4.

Bauer, R. and H. Wagner. 1991. In *Economic and Medicinal Plant Research,* v. 5. Wagner, H. & N. R. Farnsworth, eds. New York: Academic Press.

Bauer, R. 1991. Personal Communication.

Bauer, R. and S. Foster. 1991. *Planta Med.* 57: 447-9.

Bauer, R., P. Remiger, and H. Wagner. 1988a. *Dtsch. Apoth. Ztg.* 128: 174-80.

Bauer, R., P. Remiger, and H. Wagner. 1989. *Phytochemistry* 28: 505-8.

Bauer, R., P. Remiger, K. Jurcic, and H. Wagner. 1989. *Z. Phytother.* 10: 43-8.

Bauer, R. and P. Remiger. 1989b. *Planta Med.* 55: 367-71.

Bauer, R. and H. Wagner. 1987. *Sci. Pharm.* 55: 159-61.

Bauer, R., P. Remiger, V. Wray, and H. Wagner. 1988b. *Planta Med.* 54: 478-9.

Bauer, R., I. A. Khan, and H. Wagner. 1988e. *Planta Med.* 54: 426-30.

Bauer, R., K. Jurcic, J. Puhlmann,and H. Wagner. 1988d. *Arzneim.-Forsch.* 38: 276-81.

Bauer, R., I. A. Khan, and H. Wagner. 1986. *Sci. Pharm.* 54: 145.

Bauer, R. Personal communication, Jan. 19, 1993.

Becker, H. 1982. *Deut. Apoth. Zeit.* 122: 2320.

Becker, H., *et al.* 1985. *Z. Naturforsch.* 40c: 585-7.

Berkeley, E. and D. S. Berkeley. 1963. *John Clayton, Pioneer of American Botany,* University of North Carolina, p. 143.

Beuscher, H. and L. Kopanski. 1987. *Pharm. Weekbl. Sci. Ed.* 9: 329.

Bittner, E. 1969. Ph.D. Dissertation. Albert Ludwigs Universität, Freiburg.

Blake, A. K. 1929. New Asteraceae from the United States, Mexico and Honduras. *Jour. Wash. Acad. Sci.* 19: 273.

Blumenthal, M., personal communication, June 10, 1993.

Bohl, R. and T. Hermann. 1954. *Schweiz med. Wschr.* 84: 421.

Bohlmann, F. and M. Grenz. 1966. *Chem. Ber.* 99: 3197.

Bohlmann, F and H. Hoffmann. 1983. *Phytochemistry* 22: 1173.

Bonadeo, I.G., G. Botazzi, and M. Lavazza. 1971. *Riv. Ital. Essenze* 53: 281.

Bos, R., F. Heinzer, and R. Bauer. 1988. Poster, *19th International Symposium on Essential Oils and Other Natural Substrates.* Zürich, 7-10 September.

Boshamer, K. 1968. *Lehrbuch der Urologie.* Gustav Fischer Verlag, p. 74.

Bräunig, B., B. Dorn, and E. M. Knick. 1992. *Z. Phytother.* 13: 7.

Brehm, G. 1962. *Arztl. Sammelbl.* 51: 423.

Bridger, Bobby. Personal communication with Mark Blumenthal.

Britton, N. L. and A. Brown. 1896. *An Illustrated Flora of the Northern United States, Canada and the British Possessions.* NY: Charles Scribner's Sons.

Büsing, K. H. 1952. *Arzn.-Forsch.* 2: 467.

Büsing, K. H. 1958. *Z. Immunitätsforsch. Exp. Ther.* 115: 169-76.

Büsing, K. H. and G. Thüigen. 1959. *G. Allerg. Asthma* 4: 30-3.

Chamberlin, C. S. 1905. *Lancet-Clinic* n.s. 54: 279.

Cheminat, A., R. Zawatzky, H. Becker, and R. Brouillard. 1988. *Phytochemistry* 27: 2787-94.

Cheminat, A., R. Brouillard, P. Guerne, P. Bergmann, and B. Rether. 1989. *Phytochemistry* 28: 3246-7.

Choné, B. 1969. *Dt. Med. Woch.* 94: 1406.

Clayton, J. and J. F. Gronovius. 1762. *Flora Virginica*, Leiden.

Coeugniet, E. G. 1987. *Klin. Pharm.* (8/87): 481-85.

Coeugniet, E. G. and E. Elek. 1987. *Suppl. Z. Onkologie* 10: 27-33.

Coeugniet, E. and R. Kühnast. 1986. *Therapiewoche* 36: 3352.

Comings, I. M. 1847. *New. Engl. Bot. Med. Surg.* J. 1: 41.

Couch, J. F. and T. Giltner. 1921a. *Am. J. Pharm.* 93: 227.

Couch, J. F. and T. Giltner. 1921b. *Am. J. Pharm.* 93: 324.

Culter, S. H. 1930. *J. Am. Pharm. Assn.* 19: 120.

DeCandolle, A. P. and A. DeCandolle. 1824-1873. *Prodromus systematis naturalis regni vegetabilis.* 17 v. Paris.

Dorn, M. 1989. *Natur Ganzheits-Med.* 2: 314.

Dress, W. J. 1961. *Baileya* 9: 67.

Editorial. 1930. *J. Am. Pharm. Assn.* 19: 370.

Egert, D. and N. Beuscher. 1992. *Planta Med.* 58: 163.

Eilmes, H. G. 1976. Dissertation, Frankfurt.

Etsuio, B. and F. Enriko. 1992. *Jpn. Kokai Tokkyo Koho*, 5 pp. (Therapeutic extracts of *Echinacea purpurea*).

Felder, H. 1959. *Med. Klin.* 12: 525.

Fong, *et al.* 1972. *Lloydia* 35: 38.

Fontana, A. In Press. (through Schiedges, Madaus).

Foster, S. 1991. *Echinacea, Nature's Immune Enhancer.* Rochester, VT: Healing Arts Press.

Foster, S. 1985a. *Business of Herbs* 8.

Foster, S. 1985b. *HerbalGram* 3.

Franken, E. and N. Sönnichsen. 1966. *Aesthet. Medizin.* (8/66): 242-45.

Freyer, H. U. 1974. *Forschrift. der Ther.* 92: 165.

Gaertner, W. 1963. *Landarzt.* 39: 123.

Gaisbauer, M. 1990a. *Natura Med.* 5: 176-90.

Gaisbauer, M. and T. Schleich. 1986. *Natura Med.* 1: 6.

Gaisbauer, M., T. Schleich, H. A. Stickl, and I. Wilczek. 1990b. *Arzneim.-Forsch.* 40: 594-8.

Gaisbauer, M. 1990. *Natura Med.* 5: 176-90.

Gartang, E. 1993. *National Examiner*, January 12, p. 7.

Gasiorowska, I., *et al.* 1981. *Czas. Stomat.* 34: 677.

Geller, C. A. 1987. Clinical experience, personal communication.

Giesbert, M. 1943. *Fschr. Ther.* 19: 4.

Giger, E. and T.W. Baumann. 1989. *Planta Med.* 55: 638.

Gilmore, M. R. 1911. *Bur. Am. Eth. Ann. Rep.* 33, p. 368.

Gilmore, M. R. 1913. *Neb. St. Hist. Soc., Coll.* 17: 332.

Gray, A. 1848. *Manual of Botany.* Boston: James Munroe and Co.

Gray, A. 1879. *School and Field Book of Botany.* NY: Iveson, Blakeman, Taylor, p. 205.

Greger, H. 1988. In *Chemistry and Biology of Naturally Occurring Acetylenes and Related Compounds.* J. Lam, H. Breteler, T. Arnason and L. Hansen, eds., pp. 159-78. Amsterdam: Elsevier.

Gunther, E., E. F. Heeger, C. Rosenthal. 1952. *Pharmazie* 7: 24.

Hanfstaengel, E. and H. Ranz. 1956. *Zbl. Chir.*, p. 2549.

Hansen, P. 1965. *Prophylaxe* 4: 278.

Heesen, W. 1964. *Ehk* 13: 209.

Heinzer, F., M. Chavanne, J.-P. Meusy, H.-P. Maitre, E. Giger,. and T.W. Baumann. 1988. *Pharm. Acta. Helv.* 63: 132-36.

Hentges, D. J. 1983. *Human Intestinal Microflora in Health and Disease.* New York: Academic Press.

Herrmann, G. 1952. *Münch. med. Wschr.* 94: 385.

Heubl, G. R. and R. Bauer. 1988. *Sci. Pharm.* 56: 145-60.

Heubl, G. R. & R. Bauer. 1990. *Dtsch. Apoth. Ztg.* 129: 2497-99.

Heyl, F. W. and M. C. Hart. 1915. *J. Am. Chem. Soc.* 37: 1769.

Heyl, F. W. and J. F. Staley. 1914. *Am. J. Pharm.* 86: 450.

Hobbs, C. R. 1989. *The Echinacea Handbook.* Capitola: Botanica Press.

Hoh, K. 1990. Ph. D. Dissertation, Freiburg.

Höreth, W. and F. Heiss. 1957. *Medizinische,* p. 297.

Hunsdorfer, N. W. 1954. *Ärztl. Praxis* IV/8: 11.

Jacobson, M. 1954. *Science* 120: 1028.

Jacobson, M. 1967. *J. Org. Chem.* 32: 1646.

Jacobson, M. 1975. *Lloydia* 38: 473.

Jurcic, K., D. Melchart, M. Holzmann, P. Martin, R. Bauer, A. Doenicke, and H. Wagner. 1989. *Z. Phytother.* 10: 67-70.

Kelkar, P and M.A. Ross. 1994. Perspect. Biol. Med. 37: 244-6.

Kelsey, H. P. and W. A. Dayton. 1942. *Standardized Plant Names.* Harrisburg: McFarland Co.

Kennelly, J. C. 1985a. Microtest Research Ltd.: York, England.

Kennelly, J. C. 1985b. Microtest Research Ltd.: York, England.

King, J. & H. C. F. Meyer. 1887. *Eccl. Med. J.* 48: 209.

King, J. 1852. *The American Dispensatory.* Cincinnati: H.W. Derby.

Kinkel, H. J., M. Plate, and H. U. Tullner. 1984. *Med. Klin.* 79: 580.

Kleinschmidt, H. 1965. *Ther. d. Gegen.* p. 1258.

Koch, Fr. E. 1953. *Arzn.-Forsch.* 3: 16.

Koch, Fr. E. 1952. *Arzn.-Forsch.* 2: 464.

Korting, G. W. and K. Rasp. 1954. *Medizinische* 45: 1504.

Kraemer, H. and M. Sollenberger. 1911. *Am. J. Pharm.* 83: 315.

Krause, M. 1984. Dissertation, Berlin.

Krause, W. 1986. Dissertation, Tübingen.

Kuhn, O. 1953. *Arzn.-Forsch.* 3: 194.

Lang, W. and U. Mengs. 1976a. Report on Echinacea Toxicity in Mice. Cologne: Madaus GMBH.

Lang, W. and U. Mengs. 1976b. Report on Echinacea Toxicity in Rats. Cologne: Madaus GMBH., September 1, 1976.

Lasch, H. G. 1983. *Die Med. Welt.* 34: 1463.

Leng-Peschlow, E. In press, (through Schiedges, Madaus).

Lenk, W. 1989. *Z. Phytother.* 10: 49-51.

Lersch, C., *et al.* 1990a. *J. Exp. Clin. Cancer Res.* 9: 247-50.

Lersch, C., *et al.* 1990b. *Arch. Geschwulstforsch.* 60: 379-83.

Lersch, C., *et al.* 1992. *Tumordiagn. u. Ther.* 13:115-20.

Linnaeus, C. 1753. *Species Plantarum,* Vol. 2, London: Bernard Quaritch (1959), p. 907.

Lloyd, J. U. 1897. *Eccl. Med. J.* 57: 28.

Lloyd, J. U. 1904. *Pharm. Rev.* 22: 9. Reprinted by the American Herb Association, Rescue, CA.

Lloyd, J. U. 1917. *A Treatise on Echinacea.* Cincinnati: Lloyd Bros.; reprinted by Herb-Pharm, Williams, OR.

Lohamann-Matthes, M.-L., and H. Wagner. 1989. *Z. Phytother.* 10: 52-9.

Luettig, B., C. Steinmüller, G. E. Gifford, H. Wagner, and M.-L. Lomann-Matthes, 1989. *J. Natl. Cancer Inst.* 81: 669-75.

Lücker, P. W. 1982. *The Stimulant Value of Intravenous Application of Echinacea®.* Institut Für Klinische Pharmakologic, Bobenheim am Berg.

Lyons, A.B. 1907. *Plant Names, Scientific and Popular,* 2nd ed. Detroit: Nelson, Baker & Co.

Malonga-Makosi J.-P. 1983. Dissertation, University of Heidelberg.
Martin, R. 1985. Dissertation, University of Heidelberg.
May, G. and G. Willuhn. 1978. *Arzn.-Forsch.* 28: 1, 2242.
McGregor, R. L. 1968. *Univ. of Kansas Sci. Bul.* 48: 132.
Meixner, H. K. L. 1953. *Med. heute* 11: 314.
Mengs, U. 1985. Biologisches Institut Dr. Madaus GMBH & Co., Cologne.
Mengs, U., C. B. Clare, and J. A. Poiley. 1991. *Arzneim.-Forsch.* 41: 1076-81.
Miller, K. In press. (through Schiedges, Madaus).
Moench, K. 1794. *Methodas Plantas.*
Möller, H. & H. Naumann. 1987. *Therapeutikon* 1: 56-61.
Morison, R. 1699. *Plantarum Historiae Universalis Oxoniensis*, Pars tertia finished and published by Jacob Bobart the younger, p. 42.
Möse, J. R. 1983. *Die Mediz. Welt.* 34: 1463.
Moser, J. 1910. *Am. J. Pharm.* 82: 224.
Mostbeck, A. and Studlar, M. 1962. *Wiener Med. Wschr.* 112: 259.
Mund-Hoym, W.-D. 1979. *Arztl. Prax.* 31: 566.
Neugebauer, H. 1949. *Pharmazie* 4: 137.
Norton, J. B. 1902. Notes on some plants of the Southwestern United States. *Trans. Acad. Sci. St. Louis* 7: 40-41.
Nuttall, T. 1834. *J. Acad. Nat. Sci. of Phil.* 7: 77.
Nuttall, T. 1841. *Trans. Am. Phil. Soc.* n.ser. 7: 354.
Pohl, P. 1969. *Med. Klin.* 35: 1546.
Quadripur, S.-A. 1976a. *Medikamentose Beein. d. Phag. Gran.* 115: 1072.
Quadripur, S.-A. 1976b. *Ther. d. Gegen.* 115: 1072.
Rafinesque, C. S. 1830. *Medical Botany.* Philadelphia: Samuel Atkinson, p. 227.
Reissmann, G. 1966. *Folia haemotologica* 85: 125.
Reith, F. J. 1978. *Patent Ger. Offen* 2: 721: 014 through CA 90:43820t.
Remiger, P. Dissertation, University of Munich.
Reuss, D. 1981. *Z Allgemeinmed* 57: 865.
Reuss, D. 1986. *Rheuma* 5:29-32.
Riddell, J. L. 1835/6. *A Synopsis of the Flora of the Western States*, p. 58.
Robinson, H. 1978. *Phytologia* 41: 39-44.
Röder, E., *et al.* 1984. *Deut. Apoth. Zeit.* 124: 2316.
Röseler, W. 1952. *Medizinische* : 93.
Rösler, J., C. Steinmüller, A. Kinderlen, A. Emmendörffer, H. Wagner, and M.-L. Lohmann-Matthes. 1991a. *Int. J. Immunopharmacol.* 13: 27-31.
Rösler, J., Emmendörffer, Steinmüller, Luettig, B., Wagner, H. and M.-L. Lohmann-Matthes. 1991b. *Int. J. Immunopharmacol.* 13: 931-41.
Sartor, K. J. 1972. *Ther. d. Gegenw.*: 1147.
Schiedges, K. L. Madaus AG. Personal communication, May 26, 1992.
Schimmel, K. Ch., and G. T. Werner. 1981. *Ther. d. Gegen.* 120: 1065.
Schimmer, O., *et al.* 1989. *Z. Phytother.* 10: 39-42.
Schindler, H. 1953. *Arzn.-Forsch.* 3: 485.
Schmidt, U., M. Albrecht, and N. Schenk. 1990. *Natur Ganzheits-Med.* 3: 277.
Schöneberger, D. 1992. *Zeit. f. Immunologie Praxis* (*Forum Immunologie* 8: 2-12.).
Schranner, I., Würdinger, N. Klumpp, U. Lösch and S. N. Okpanyi. 1989. *J. Vet. Med.* B 36: 353-64.
Schulte, K. E., G. Ruecker, and J. Perlick. 1967. *Arzn.-Forsch.* 17: 825-29.
Schulthess, B. H., E. R. Giger, and T. W. Baumann. 1988. Poster, *36th Annual Congress of the Society of Medicinal Plant Research*, Freiburg, 12-16 September.
Schulthess, B. H., E. Giger, and T.W. Baumann. 1991. *Planta Med.* 57: 384-8.
Schumacher, A. and K.-K. Friedberg. 1991. *Arzneim.-Forsch.* 41: 141-7.
Schuster, A. 1952. *Med. Mschr.* 6: 453.

Sícha, J., J. Hubík, and J. Dusek. 1989. *Ceskoslov. Farm. 38: 128-9*.
Sícha, J., H. Becker, J. Dusek, T. Hubík, J. Siatka and I. Hrones. 1991. *Pharmazie* 46: 363-4.
Sickel, K. 1971. *Ärztl. Prax.* 23: 201.
Small, J. K. 1933. *Manual of the Southeastern Flora.* Chapel Hill: Univ. of N.C. Press.
Soicke, H., K. Görler, and D. Krüger. 1988. *Fitoterapiea* 59: 73-5.
Sprockhoff, O. 1964. *Landarzt* 40: 1173.
Sprockhoff, O. 1986. *Ärztezeit. f. Naturheil.* 27: 780.
Stimpel, M., A. Proksch, H. Wagner, and M.L. Lohmann-Matthes. 1984. *Inf. and Immun.* 46: 845.
Stites, D. P., J. D. Stobo, H. H. Fudenberg, and J.V. Wells. 1982. *Basic and Clinical Immunology* (4th ed.). Los Altos, CA: Lange Medical Publications.
Stoll, A., J. Renz and A. Brack. 1950. *Helv. Chim. Acta* 33: 1877.
Stotzem, C. D., U. Hungerland. and U. Mengs. 1992. *Med. Sci. Res.* 20: 719.
Stuessy, T F. 1977. In *The Biology and Chemistry of the Compositae* ed. V. H. Harborne, J.B. Harborne and B. L. Turner, Vol. II, pp. 622-671. London: Academic Press.
Stuppner, H. 1985. Ph.D. Dissertation, Ludwig-Maximillians-Universität, München.
Thackeray, W. T. 1923. *Am. J. Clin. Med.* 30: 430.
Tosetti, K. 1961. *Dtsch. Gesuhdb.-Wes.* 16: 64.
Tronnier, H. 1967. *Munch. med. Wschr.* 109: 2118.
Tubaro, A., *et al.* 1987. *J. Pharm. Pharmacol.* 39: 567.
Tympner, K.-D. 1978. *Münch. med. Wschr.* 120: 1055.
Tympner, K.-D., P. K. Klose and R. B. Pelka. 1987. *Natura Med.* 2: 78-84.
Uhlmann, W.-J. 1958. *Medizinische* 2: 81-4.
Unruh, V. 1915. *Nat. Eclec. Med. Assn. Q.* 7: 63.
Verelis, C. and H. Becker. 1977. *Planta Med.* 31: 288.
Verelis, C. 1978. Dissertation, University of Heidelberg.
Viehmann, P. 1978. *Erhahrungsheilkunde* 27: 353.
Voaden, D.J. and M. Jacobson. 1972. *J. Med. Chem.* 15: 619.
Vogel, G. *et al.* 1968. *Arzn.-Forsch.* 18: 426.
Vogel V. 1977. *American Indian Medicine,* Norman, Oklahoma. University of Oklahoma Press.
Volz, G. 1957. *Ther. Ggw.* 96: 312.
Vömel, T. 1985. *Arzn.-Forsch.* 35: 1437.
Vorberg, G. and B. Schneider. 1989. *Ärztl. Fortschr.* 36: 3.
Wacker, A., *et al.* 1973. *Arzneim.-Forsch.* 23: 119.
Wacker, A. and A. Hilbig. 1978. *Planta Med.* 33: 89.
Wagner, H., H. Stuppner, J. Puhlmann, B. Brümmer, K. Deppe, and M.A. Zenk. 1989. *Z. Phytother.* 10: 35-8.
Wagner, H., A. Proksch, *et al.* 1981. *Z. für Angewandte Phytotherapie* 2: 166.
Wagner, H and A. Proksch. 1985a. In: *Economic and Medicinal Plant Research.* Orlando: Academic Press, p. 113.
Wagner, H. and K. Jurcic. 1991. *Arzn.-Forsch.* 41: 1072-6.
Webster, H. T. 1891. *Massachusetts Medical J.* 11: 344.
Wedel, W. 1936. *Bur. Am. Ethn. Bull.* 112: 59.
Weissbach, L ., *et al.* 1977. *Therapiewoche* 27: 6009.
Wember, S. 1953. *Landarzt.* 29: 621.
Wood -. 1925. *Propagateur de l'Homeopathie.*
Woods, E. L. 1930. *Am. J. Pharm.* 102: 611-630.
Zimmermann, O. 1969. *Hippokrates* 40: 233.

Author's Disclaimer.

The information given in this book is for educational purposes and is not meant as a prescription for any ailment. If you have a serious illness, the author recommends seeking the services of a competent natural health practitioner. Unless a statement is specifically referenced, it could be the author's opinion, based on extensive study and personal experience.